Practical Guide for Imaging of Soft Tissue Tumours

Soft tissue tumours are extremely common, but are difficult to understand due to a large number of subtypes, leading to a significant increase in their imaging in the past decade. This highly illustrated practical book provides a simplified, systematic approach to imaging, reporting and diagnosing these tumours. It covers all the modalities with emphasis on ultrasound and magnetic resonance imaging (MRI), along with the newer techniques in these modalities. This concise guide to soft tissue lesions will help clinicians to quickly understand the spectrum of tumours and identify the appropriate imaging techniques to best serve their patients.

Key features:

- Provides guidance by international experts on various types of soft tissue tumours (benign, malignant and tumour mimics), their relevant imaging features to help suggest specific or differential diagnosis, and when to biopsy and when to refer to specialist centres.
- Proves to be an excellent resource for general and specialist radiologists, radiology trainees, sonographers, sarcoma surgeons and oncologists for day-to-day reporting.
- Discusses the importance of proper imaging and biopsy of tumours and the implications of unplanned excisions in sarcoma.

Practical Guide for Imaging of Soft Tissue Tumours

Edited by

Harun Gupta MBBS, MD, DNB, MRCP (UK), FRCR (UK)
Consultant Musculoskeletal Radiologist
Leeds Teaching Hospitals

Siddharth Thaker MBBS, MD (India), FRCR (UK)
Consultant Musculoskeletal Radiologist
University Hospitals of Leicester NHS Trust

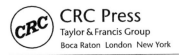

CRC Press
Taylor & Francis Group
Boca Raton London New York

CRC Press is an imprint of the
Taylor & Francis Group, an **informa** business

First edition published 2023
by CRC Press
6000 Broken Sound Parkway NW, Suite 300, Boca Raton, FL 33487-2742

and by CRC Press
4 Park Square, Milton Park, Abingdon, Oxon, OX14 4RN

CRC Press is an imprint of Taylor & Francis Group, LLC

ISBN: 978-1-032-11176-6 (hbk)
ISBN: 978-1-032-11175-9 (pbk)
ISBN: 978-1-003-21872-2 (ebk)

DOI: 10.1201/9781003218722

Typeset in Gill Sans
by KnowledgeWorks Global Ltd.

*To my dear parents, Vimla and Chittaranjan, and my wife Olivia
and daughters Alysha and Jasmine, for their constant encouragement,
love and support.*

Dr Harun Gupta

*To my parents – Narendrabhai and Jyotiben – and my partner Kanika,
for their altruistic support and love. To my teachers, colleagues and friends
who have constantly inspired me.*

Dr Siddharth Thaker

Contents

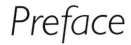 # Preface

Soft tissue lesions, sometimes referred to as "lumps and bumps", are very common in clinical practice. These have seen an increase in their imaging due to improved public awareness and advances in imaging. However, the vast number of different types of soft tissue tumours and their mimics makes their diagnosis challenging. Imaging plays a vital role in their management from diagnosis or differential diagnosis to biopsy, staging and post-treatment follow up.

Our book has been written with the aim of providing radiologists, including those under training, sonographers and sarcoma clinicians, with a handy guide covering various subtypes of soft tissue tumours as per the latest WHO classification, and simplifying approach and understanding of these lesions. The book also has chapters covering soft tissue tumour biopsy, histopathology, post-treatment imaging and soft tissue tumour mimics.

All the chapters illustrate the lesions with example images covering different modalities. These include ultrasound, MRI including advanced sequences, computed tomography and positron emission tomography-CT. Charts and flow charts have been used extensively throughout the book and each chapter has "Take-Home Points" in the end.

We would like to thank all the authors who have contributed chapters to this book and thank the publishers for all their help at every stage of the publication. We would like to particularly thank Himani Dwivedi and Shivangi Pramanik for their tireless efforts and for putting up with us through the editorial process.

Dr Harun Gupta
Dr Siddharth Thaker

About the editors

Harun Gupta

Dr Gupta is consultant musculoskeletal radiologist at Leeds Teaching Hospitals since 2010. He did his radiology training from Aberdeen and also did out-of-program training in Oxford, which was followed by 1-year MSK Fellowship in Leeds. He is expert in all aspects of musculoskeletal radiology with subspecialty interests in soft tissue sarcoma and musculoskeletal intervention. He is elected member of the Council, British Society of Skeletal Radiology (BSSR); advisory editor, MSK Section, *Clinical Radiology Journal*; member of the Ultrasound and Intervention sub-committees, European Society of Skeletal Radiology (ESSR); member of Refresher Program Promotion Committee, International Skeletal Society (ISS); advisory member of the Board, MSK Society of India; and honorary senior lecturer, University of Leeds, UK.

He is actively involved in training the specialist registrars and the MSK radiology fellows. He has been the Special Interest Lead for MSK for the Leeds Radiology Academy and Clinical Supervisor for all the trainees in MSK department. He also helped the RCR with Making Best Use of Radiology Department (iRefer) as the Lead for the MSK Sub-section.

He has more than 55 publications in peer-reviewed journals and book chapters. He regularly contributes to teaching through lectures, courses and webinars at national and international levels. He is also actively involved in research at the NIHR Leeds Biomedical Research Centre.

Siddharth Thaker

Dr Thaker is a dual fellowship-trained consultant musculoskeletal radiologist currently working at the University Hospitals of Leicester NHS Trust. He has completed his general radiology residency in India which was followed by a year-long musculoskeletal fellowship in Mumbai under mentorship of Dr Daftary. Having obtained FRCR qualification in 2018, he moved to the UK to further his academic career and completed an extended musculoskel-etal radiology fellowship at Leeds in 2022.

He is a proud recipient of the prestigious ESOR scholarship with which he has attended Medical University of Vienna enhancing his skills especially in fields of advances in musculo-skeletal radiology and research. He enjoys all facets of musculoskeletal radiology including soft tissue sarcoma imaging, musculoskeletal interventions, rheumatology, spinal imaging and musculoskeletal trauma. He is a member of multiple societies contributing to the subject including BSSR, ESSR, ECR, RSNA, MSS (India), IRIA and KSUM and is also an active member of an exclusive ESSR young club.

He is particularly passionate about musculoskeletal radiology research and education. He regularly contributes to undergraduate and registrar teaching using various online platforms and in-person basis. He is a well-published author with 22 publications in peer-reviewed indexed journals and a reviewer for *IJRI, AJR*, clinical radiology and tomography journals. He is a regular speaker in India and UK based conferences. He believes in continuous and unhindered propagation of musculoskeletal radiology education and makes constant efforts to achieve this goal.

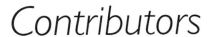# Contributors

Ankita Ahuja
Consultant Musculoskeletal Radiologist
Innovision Imaging
Mumbai, India

Hayder Al-Assam
Specialist Trainee in Radiology
Royal Orthopaedic Hospital
Birmingham, United Kingdom

Ehsan Alipour
Division of Musculoskeletal Imaging and Intervention
Department of Radiology & Department of Biomedical Informatics and Medical Education
University of Washington
Seattle, Washington

Oganes Ashikyan
Division of Musculoskeletal Imaging
Department of Radiology
University of Texas Southwestern Medical Center
Dallas, Texas

Abhinav Bansal
Fellow, Diagnostic and Interventional GI Radiology
Department of Radio Diagnosis & Interventional Radiology
All India Institute of Medical Sciences (AIIMS)
New Delhi, India

Rajesh Botchu
Consultant Musculoskeletal Radiologist
Royal Orthopaedic Hospital
Birmingham, United Kingdom.

Nivedita Chakrabarty
Assistant Professor and Consultant Radiologist
Tata Memorial Hospital
Tata Memorial Center
Dr Homi Bhabha National Institute (HBNI)
Mumbai, India

Majid Chalian
Division of Musculoskeletal Imaging and Intervention
Department of Radiology
University of Washington
Seattle, Washington

Aditya Daftary
Consultant Musculoskeletal Radiologist
Innovision Imaging
Mumbai, India

Sara Edward
Consultant Histopathologist
Leeds Teaching Hospitals NHS Trust
Leeds, United Kingdom

Ankur Goyal
Additional Professor and Consultant Radiologist
Department of Radio Diagnosis & Interventional Radiology
All India Institute of Medical Sciences (AIIMS)
New Delhi, India

Moomal Rose Haris
Consultant Radiologist
Department of Radiology
Calderdale and Huddersfield Foundation NHS Trust
Huddersfield, United Kingdom

Ganesh Hegde
Locum Consultant Radiologist
University Hospitals of Morecambe Bay NHS Foundation Trust
Lancaster, United Kingdom

Slavcho Ivanoski
St. Erazmo Hospital for Orthopaedic Surgery and Traumatology
Ohrid, North Macedonia

Karthikeyan P Iyengar
Department of Trauma and Orthopaedics
Southport and Ormskirk NHS Trust
Southport, United Kingdom

Malini Lawande
Consultant Musculoskeletal Radiologist
Innovision Imaging
Mumbai, India

Ajay Maliyakkal
Consultant Musculoskeletal Radiologist
University Hospitals of Leicester NHS Trust
Leicester, United Kingdom

Ramy Mansour
Consultant Musculoskeletal Radiologist
Radiology Department
Nuffield Orthopaedic Centre
Oxford University Hospitals NHS Trust
Oxford, United Kingdom

Asimenia Mermekli
Radiology Department
John Radcliffe Hospital
Oxford University Hospitals NHS Trust
Oxford, United Kingdom

Violeta Vasilevska Nikodinovska
Professor of Radiology
Subspecialist in Musculoskeletal Radiology
University 'Ss.Cyril and Methodius' in Skopje
Faculty of Medicine
University Institute of Radiology
Clinical Center 'Mother Theresa'
Skopje, North Macedonia

Parham Pezeshk
Division of Musculoskeletal Imaging
Department of Radiology
University of Texas Southwestern Medical Center
Dallas, Texas

Niharika Prasad
Consultant Radiologist
Department of Radiology
IOCL Hospital
Barauni, India

Winston Rennie
Consultant Musculoskeletal Radiologist
University Hospitals of Leicester NHS Trust
Leicester, United Kingdom

Amit Shah
Consultant Musculoskeletal Radiologist
University Hospitals of Leicester NHS Trust
Leicester, United Kingdom

Sandeep Singh Sidhu
Musculoskeletal Radiology Fellow
Radiology Department
Nuffield Orthopaedic Centre
Oxford University Hospitals NHS Trust
Oxford, United Kingdom

Jordan ZT Sim
Department of Diagnostic Radiology
Tan Tock Seng Hospital
Singapore, Singapore

Ankit A Tandon
Consultant Musculoskeletal Radiologist
Department of Diagnostic Radiology
Tan Tock Seng Hospital
Singapore, Singapore

Aanand Vibhakar
Specialist Trainee in Radiology (ST5)
University Hospitals of Leicester NHS Trust
Leicester, United Kingdom

Approach to soft tissue lesions

Moomal Rose Haris, Niharika Prasad, Harun Gupta

INTRODUCTION

Soft tissue lesions are a heterogeneous group of lesions ranging from benign to malignant lesions, including soft tissue tumour mimics. Soft tissue lesions arise from mesenchymal tissues such as fat, muscle, nerves, blood vessels and fibrous tissue. These are immensely common in clinical practice, and the majority of these are benign. In contrast, soft tissue sarcomas are uncommon and account for less than 1% of all adult malignancies. It is believed that a general practitioner may only see one case in their working lifetime. However, delayed initiation of treatment for soft tissue sarcomas is associated with poor clinical outcomes, with a 5-year survival rate of around 50%.

Trends in the imaging of soft tissue lesions have been changing with time. There has been a gradual evolution from relying on plain radiographs and computed tomography (CT) to ultrasound (US) and magnetic resonance imaging (MRI). Imaging plays a significant role in the diagnosis and biopsy of soft tissue lesions along with staging and post-treatment follow-up of proven soft tissue sarcoma.

There is a need for a systematic approach to classifying and diagnosing soft tissue tumours and tumour-like lesions. Clinical history, lesion location, lesion borders, mineralisation on radiographs, sonographic appearances including Doppler flow and signal characteristics on MRI are all essential to form a diagnosis or at least a limited differential list. Imaging often allows the lesion to be categorised as benign, malignant or indeterminate. Despite advancements in imaging techniques, it is usually only possible to make a definitive imaging diagnosis in one-quarter to one-third of cases, and many remain indeterminate. Often the benign lesions of different subtypes have more typical imaging appearances (Figure 1.1). The indeterminate and malignant lesions require further workup, usually starting with a biopsy.

WORLD HEALTH ORGANIZATION (WHO) CLASSIFICATION

The WHO classification of soft tissue tumours is the most widely and commonly accepted pathology-based classification system for such disorders. At the time of publishing, the most up-to-date WHO classification of soft tissue tumours was developed in 2020 and represented the fifth edition in this series.

Significant changes within the fifth edition of the WHO classification include greater awareness and understanding of the importance of molecular genetic characterisation, novel

DOI: 10.1201/9781003218722-1

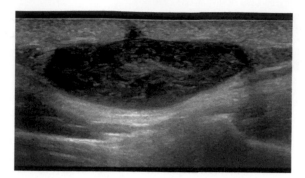

Figure 1.1: Epidermal inclusion cyst. Ultrasound demonstrates a well-circumscribed, ovoid, predominantly hypoechoic mass. Located close to the skin surface with characteristic tract seen extending to the skin surface.

ancillary diagnostic tests and new disease entities such as undifferentiated small round cell sarcomas of bone and soft tissues and overall refinements in tumour classification (Table 1.1).

Histopathology remains the gold standard for diagnosing and grading soft tissue tumours. However, radiology–pathology correlation is still crucial to prevent any diagnostic pitfalls. In addition to lesion localisation, characterisation, staging and follow-up, imaging allows differentiation from tumour-like lesions such as haematomas, abscess, myositis and ganglia, to name a few.

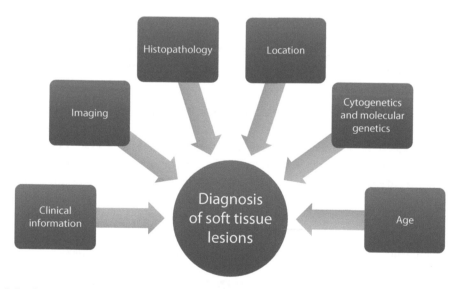

Chart 1.1: Overview of various components involved in the diagnosis of soft tissue lesions

CLINICAL EVALUATION

Clinicians want the radiologist to confirm the presence of the lesion, characterise it anatomically with all its relations and give a definitive or differential diagnosis. Table 1.2 lists the important clinical questions to help aid the radiologist in prioritising the patient and forming a diagnosis.

Table 1.1: Selected Soft Tissue Tumour Categories Based on WHO Classification

	Lipomatous	Vascular	Fibrous	Muscle	Neural	Unknown differentiation
Benign	Lipoma Lipoma variants	Haemangioma	Nodular fasciitis Elastofibroma	Leiomyoma rhabdomyoma	Schwannoma Neurofibroma	Myxoma
Locally aggressive	Atypical lipomatous tumour		Solitary fibrous tumour Fibromatosis			
Rarely metastatic		Kaposi's sarcoma	Dermatofibrosarcoma protuberans (DFSP) (Figure 1.2) Solitary fibrous tumour Myxoinflammatory fibroblastic sarcoma			
Malignant	Liposarcoma (well-differentiated Myxoid Dedifferentiated, pleomorphic)	Angiosarcoma	Solitary fibrous tumour Fibrosarcoma Myxofibrosarcoma	Leiomyosarcoma Rhabdomyosarcoma	Malignant peripheral nerve sheath tumour (MPNST)	Synovial sarcoma Epithelioid sarcoma Undifferentiated pleomorphic sarcoma Undifferentiated spindle cell sarcoma

Soft tissue lesions

Table 1.2: **Pertinent Clinical Questions**

Clinical questions to ask the patient	Relevance
Painful or asymptomatic	Painful lesions are more concerning but this may be due to pressure effect. An asymptomatic lesion does not always indicate benignity.
Increase in size (rapid or slow)	Slow increase in size is often less concerning than rapid increase.
Lesion size	Lesions greater than 5 cm are more concerning for malignancy.
Solitary or multiple lesions	Multiple lesions do not always mean malignancy (Figure 1.3) but the metastatic disease should be considered. Multiple soft tissue lesions can be seen as part of other conditions (e.g. Cowden's syndrome, familial multiple lipomatosis [FML]).
Lesion location	Certain lesions are known to occur more commonly or exclusively at certain locations (e.g. elastofibroma, Figure 1.4). Lesions deep to the fascia are more concerning for sinister pathology.
Lesion borders	Ill-defined lesions are more concerning for malignancy compared to well-defined/encapsulated lesions.
History of prior or current malignancy +/- resection	History or current malignancy is concerning with a new-onset soft tissue lesion.

NATIONAL INSTITUTE OF CLINICAL EXCELLENCE (NICE) UK GUIDELINES

NICE guidelines regarding sarcoma evaluation recommend that all patients with bone or soft tissue sarcomas have their management care plan confirmed by a sarcoma multidisciplinary team (MDT) and treatment delivered by services designated by this sarcoma MDT. Patients with suspected sarcoma should be imaged and reviewed within two weeks.

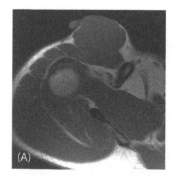 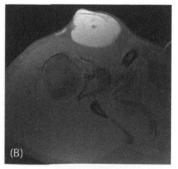

Figure 1.2: (A and B) Dermatofibrosarcoma protruberans (DFSP). T1-weighted and fluid-sensitive MRI demonstrating a well-defined mass lesion within the dermal and subcutaneous tissues. The lesion is generally of low signal on T1-weighted imaging (as in this case) and hyperintense on T2-weighted and fluid-sensitive imaging.

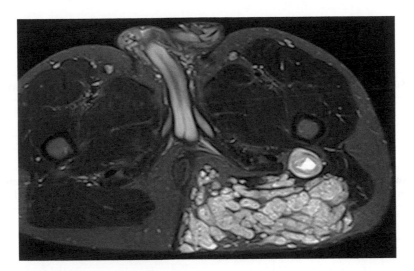

Figure 1.3: Multiple neurofibromas seen at the left buttock. Fluid-sensitive MRI demonstrates multiple, predominantly ovoid shaped high signal intensity lesions some of which demonstrate characteristic target sign.

Given the above, radiologists in a non-specialist set-up should be aware of local and regional guidelines for sarcoma MDT referral for indeterminate and malignant soft tissue lesions. Flowchart 1.1 shows a basic guideline to give an idea of the referral pathway.

IMAGING MODALITIES

The choices of imaging modalities available for soft tissue lesion evaluation have changed and progressed. However, the main objectives of imaging to get a diagnosis and staging remain the same. Often imaging modalities can be complementary to one another and a combination is needed to reach a differential or a definitive diagnosis.

● *Radiographs*

These are an inexpensive first-line imaging modality for assessing soft tissue lesions, especially extremity lesions. Radiographs can show bone lesions that may mimic soft tissue lesions

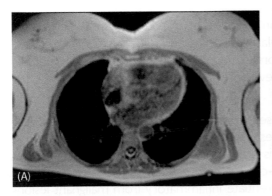
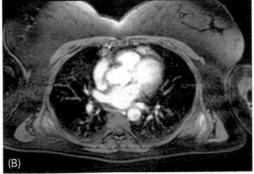

Figure 1.4: (A and B) Bilateral elastofibromas. T1-weighted and fluid-sensitive MRI sequences. Typical infrascapular location with alternating fibrous and fatty components evident.

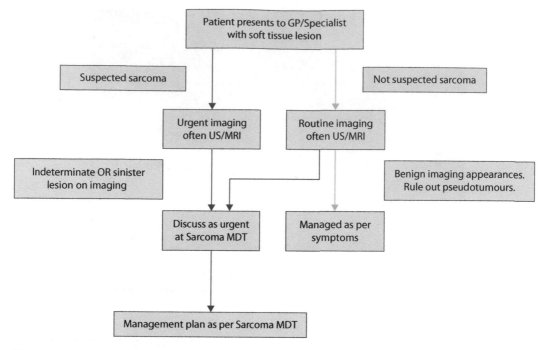

Flowchart 1.1: **Soft tissue tumour evaluation basic pathway**

(e.g. osteochondroma), areas of mineralisation (e.g. phleboliths, myositis ossificans, tumoral calcinosis) and any co-existent bone involvement.

● *Ultrasound*

US is another inexpensive and non-invasive imaging modality that assesses superficial soft tissue lesions. It enables solid masses to be differentiated from cystic masses and allows for vascular flow evaluation through Doppler imaging. Solid lesions with vascularity are more concerning than cystic avascular lesions. Ultrasound has the added benefit of not using ionising radiation, so it can be used in the paediatric population and as follow-up for many lesions.

● *Computed tomography*

CT can provide more detail regarding a lesion's mineralisation pattern, density pattern(e.g. fat), co-existent bone involvement and vascularity patterns if intravenous contrast is used. CT is more accessible than MRI and is often preferred in patients who cannot tolerate MRI due to claustrophobia or MRI-incompatible devices (e.g. cardiac pacemakers).

Positron emission tomography

The most common radioisotope currently used for positron emission tomography (PET) is fluoro-2-deoxy-glucose (FDG). FDG behaves like glucose within the body and is used to quantify glucose metabolism. PET-CT imaging is already established for the staging of various malignancies, including lymphomas, non-small-cell lung cancer and head and neck cancers. Pitfalls for PET-CT include its inability to differentiate inflammatory from malignant lesions, both of which utilise FDG. PET-CT is still under evaluation for its utility in soft tissue tumour evaluation and staging, but it is gaining popularity in the research phase.

● *Magnetic resonance imaging*

This is the preferred imaging modality for evaluating deep and/or large soft tissue lesions. MRI has superior soft tissue contrast resolution capability compared to the other imaging modalities. Optimising imaging protocol for assessing soft tissue lesions (e.g. T1-weighted, fluid-sensitive, gradient echo, diffusion-weighted imaging) using surface markers and coils enables diagnostic certainty in several conditions (e.g. lipomatous lesions, PVNS). There are contradictory views regarding the use of contrast in soft tissue evaluation. Still, intravenous contrast can help characterise certain lesions (e.g. nerve sheath tumours) and differentiate cystic from solid areas.

APPROACH TO SOFT TISSUE LESIONS

As mentioned in the chapter, definitive diagnosis based on imaging alone can be reached in only about one-fourth to one-third of cases. A systematic approach makes a significant improvement in diagnosis. This involves:

- Review of the imaging features – US and MRI
- Anatomic location of the lesion
- Age of the patient
- Multiplicity of the lesions
- Clinical history – growth of lesion over time

Ultrasound features such as hypoechoic pattern, irregular margin and increased vascularisation are more predictive of malignancy. Some superficial lesions have recognised ultrasound features of a specific tumour type (such as lipoma, nerve sheath tumour, haemangioma) and absence of such typical appearances would put the lesion in the indeterminate or aggressive category, needing further characterisation and definitive diagnosis.

MRI involves assessing for signs, signal characteristics (Table 1.3) and morphology of lesions. Differentiating benign and malignant tumours based on MRI is not straightforward as no features can be said to be completely specific for malignancy. Suspicious characteristics for malignancy are ill-defined margins, extra compartmental extension, inhomogeneity on all pulse sequences, intralesional necrosis and bone or neurovascular involvement.

Table 1.3: **Signal Pattern on MRI**

Signal pattern	MRI T1-weighted sequence	MRI T2-weighted sequence
Lipomatous lesion	Hyperintense	Hyperintense
Subacute haematoma Haemangioma Neurogenic tumour	Intermediate	Hyperintense
Myxoma Cyst Myxoid liposarcoma	Hypointense	Hyperintense
Desmoid/Fibromatosis PVNS/giant cell tumour Myositis ossificans	Hypointense	Hypointense

Table 1.4: Location Approach

Location clues	Differentials
Subungual	Glomus tumours
Intra-articular	Synovial-based pathology (e.g. haemangioma, PVNS, lipoma arborescens)
Subscapular	Elastofibroma
Achilles tendon related	Xanthoma
Tendon	Giant cell tumour of tendon sheath (Figure 1.5)
Abdominal wall	Desmoid (Figure 1.6)
Subcutaneous layer	Lipoma, nodular fasciitis, myxofibrosarcoma, dermatofibrosarcoma protruberans (Figure 1.2)
Course of major nerves	Nerve sheath tumours

Location of the soft tissue tumours can sometimes provide a clue to their diagnosis (Table 1.4).

With regards to **age**, common soft tissue tumours in the paediatric population include:

- Haemangiomas
- Lipoblastoma
- Fibrous hamartoma
- Granuloma annulare
- Rhabdomyosarcoma

Listed below are the conditions known to present with **multiple** soft tissue lesions:

- Lipomas
- Neural lesions – neurofibromatosis, schwannomatosis

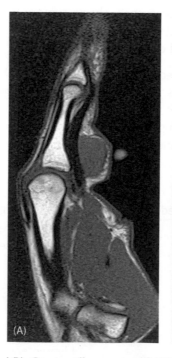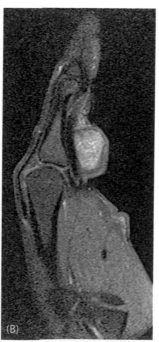

Figure 1.5: **(A and B) Giant cell tumour (GCT) arising from flexor tendon sheath at level of proximal interphalangeal joint. T1-weighted and fluid-sensitive sequences demonstrate low and heterogenous high signal, respectively.**

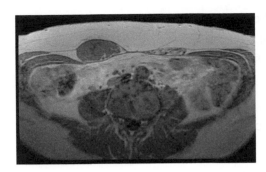

Figure 1.6: Desmoid tumour. T1-weighted MRI sequence. Common location of desmoid tumour in the abdominal wall. Low signal intensity on T1- and T2-weighted imaging secondary to dense internal cellularity.

- Vascular
  - Benign (haemangioma, lymphangioma)
  - Malignant (angiosarcoma)
- Fibromatosis
- Metastases

Finally, **typical signs** associated with certain soft tissue tumours are as follows:
- *Neural:* Target sign (central low signal surrounded by a high signal on T2W MRI)
- *Synovial sarcoma:* triple sign (areas of low, intermediate and high signal on T2W MRI)
- *Myxoma:* Bright cap sign (rim of fat at the superior and inferior pole of the lesion and surrounding oedema due to leakage of myxomatous tissue)
- *Undifferentiated pleomorphic sarcoma, myxofibrosarcoma:* Tail sign (tapering marginal extension along the fascia)

American Joint Committee on Cancer (AJCC) classification is widely followed for staging of soft tissue sarcomas and this takes into consideration TNM and histologic grading. (Table 1.5)

Table 1.5: AJCC TNM Classification for Soft Tissue Sarcoma

Classification	Description
Primary tumour (T)	
T1a	Superficial tumour ≤5 cm in greatest dimension
T1b	Deep tumour ≤5 cm in greatest dimension
T2a	Superficial tumour >5 cm in greatest dimension
T2b	Deep tumour >5 cm in greatest dimension
Regional lymph nodes (N)	
N0	No regional lymph node metastasis
N1	Regional lymph node metastasis
Distant metastasis (M)	
M0	No distant metastasis
M1	Distant metastasis
Histologic grade (G)	
G1	Well-differentiated
G2	Moderately differentiated
G3	Poorly differentiated

Table 1.6: **Soft Tissue Lesion Reporting Template**

- Confirm presence of the lesion
  - Size (in three planes)
  - Number
- Location
  - Subcutaneous
  - Deep-seated – subfascial, muscular compartment
  - Relations
- Imaging characteristics
- Diagnosis
  - Specific diagnosis/differential diagnosis
  - Indeterminate/aggressive
  - Referral to a specialist centre

REPORTING TEMPLATE

Table 1.6 is a model soft tissue reporting template which will allow consistency and quality when faced with such lesions.

CONCLUSION

This chapter serves as an introduction to the evaluation of soft tissue tumours. The radiologist should determine the tissue from which the lesion is arising (e.g. fat, fibrous, nerve, synovial or vascular). A systematic approach covering the imaging, anatomical location, age of the patient, and clinical history of pain and size of the lesion over a period helps significantly improve the diagnosis or limit the differential diagnosis. The book covers the main aspects of the latest WHO classification of soft tissue tumours. A multidisciplinary and patient-centred approach is recommended and should be employed to reach a diagnosis and an agreed management plan.

SUGGESTED READING

- Aga, P, Singh, R, Parihar, A, Parashari, U. Imaging spectrum in soft tissue sarcomas. Indian J Surg Oncol. 2011;2(4): 271–279. doi: 10.1007/s13193-011-0095-1.
- Caracciolo, JT, Letson, GD. Radiologic approach to bone and soft tissue sarcomas. Surg Clin North Am. 2016 Oct;96(5):963–976. doi: 10.1016/j.suc.2016.05.007.
- Choi, JH, Ro, JY. The 2020 WHO classification of tumors of soft tissue: Selected changes and new entities. Adv Anat Pathol. 2021 Jan;28(1):44–58. doi: 10.1097/PAP.0000000000000284.
- Dangoor, A, Seddon, B, Gerrand, C et al. UK guidelines for the management of soft tissue sarcomas. Clin Sarcoma Res. 2016 6:20. doi: https://doi.org/10.1186/s13569-016-0060-4.
- Edge, SB, Byrd, DR, Compton, CC, et al. (editors). AJCC cancer staging manual. 7th ed. New York: Springer; 2010, p. 291–298.
- Gómez, J, Tsagozis, P. Multidisciplinary treatment of soft tissue sarcomas: An update. World J Clin Oncol. 2020;11(4):180–189. doi: 10.5306/wjco.v11.i4.180.
- Grimer, RJ. Size matters for sarcomas! Ann R Coll Surg Engl. 2006;88(6):519–524. doi: 10.1308/003588406X130651.
- Hung, EHY et al. Ultrasound of musculoskeletal soft-tissue tumors superficial to the investing fascia. AJR Am J Roentgenol. 2014 Jun;202:W532. http://dx.doi.org/10.2214/AJR.13.11457.

- Hung, EH, Griffith, JF, Ng, AW, Lee, RK, Lau, DT, Leung, JC. Ultrasound of musculoskeletal soft-tissue tumors superficial to the investing fascia. AJR Am J Roentgenol. 2014 Jun;202(6):W532–W540. doi: 10.2214/AJR.13.11457.
- Kransdorf, MJ, Murphey, MD. Imaging of soft tissue tumors. 3rd ed. Philadelphia, PA: Lippincott Williams and Wilkins; (1 Oct. 2013)
- National Institute for Health and Care Excellence. Sarcoma. 29/01/2015. Quality standard SQ78. https://www.nice.org.uk/guidance/qs78
- Vadapalli, R, Hegde, G, Botchu, R MRI imaging of soft tissues tumours and tumour like lesions-SLAM approach. J Clin Orthop Trauma. 2022 Apr 16;28:101872. doi: 10.1016/j.jcot.2022.101872.

2 Imaging modalities and techniques in soft tissue tumours

Violeta Vasilevska Nikodinovska,
Slavcho Ivanoski

INTRODUCTION

Suspected soft tissue sarcomas require a systemic approach combining thorough clinical and imaging investigations simultaneously. A review of previous investigations and imaging, as well as clinical details, such as duration and rapidity of the growth, skin changes and tenderness, may give information narrowing the differential diagnosis.

Imaging evaluation often starts with an ultrasound (US) examination, which is considered as the initial modality of choice for visible and palpable soft tissue lesions. It gives sufficient information about tissue structure, allowing differentiation of benign and tumour-like lesions from malignant lesions in many cases. Power Doppler imaging can demonstrate tumour vascularity. Magnetic resonance imaging (MRI) is the modality of choice for soft tissue tumour imaging due to its multiplanar capabilities and high contrast resolution. Computed tomography is predominantly used for staging sarcomas and in cases where MRI is contraindicated.

IMAGING MODALITIES

● Ultrasound

US is the first-line imaging method for suspected soft tissue lesions following the clinical examination. The particular role of US is to detect and confirm the presence of soft tissue lesions and offer characterisation and specific diagnosis where possible. It is accurate for differentiating benign from malignant superficial soft tissue lesions. Large-sized lesions (>5 cm) with deep location, rapid growth and disorganised vascularity on Doppler US suggest aggressive behaviour or malignancy (Figure 2.1).

Technical considerations:

- It should be ideally performed using a high-frequency linear transducer (>9–18 MHz).
- Avoid pressure on superficial lesions and use the "gel stand-off" technique.
- Curved-array transducers can be used to evaluate the masses with deeper locations with a large field of view (FOV).
- In addition, panoramic US and extended FOV can be used for assessment (has no role in staging large or deep tumours).

DOI: 10.1201/9781003218722-2

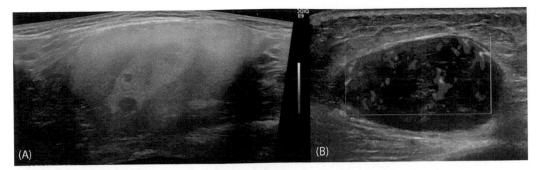

Figure 2.1: Ultrasound features of aggressive soft tissue lesions: Panoramic grey scale image (A) through the lesion in the left distal thigh demonstrates a large, deep, predominantly fatty lesion within the posterior thigh compartment muscles with internal round echo poor foci. The ultrasound appearances are very suspicious for aggressive lipomatous lesion (proven myxoid liposarcoma), and colour Doppler (B) image through a well-defined, rapidly enlarging mass overlying the right tibial shin demonstrates disorganised internal vascularity (biopsy proven undifferentiated pleomorphic sarcoma). (Image Courtesy of Dr. Harun Gupta.)

Uses of the ultrasound:

- Anatomical location may suggest the diagnosis (ganglia, Baker cyst, peripheral nerve sheath tumour, Morel-Lavallee lesions, juxta-articular cysts and pseudoaneurysm).
- Sonographic assessment of the extension, size, shape, number of lesions, location, nature (solid versus cystic), vascularity, depth, and anatomical relationship to investing fascia, neurovascular structures, and other adjacent structures (tendon and tendon sheath, joints) should aid in lesion characterisation and determine the need for further imaging or biopsy.
- Tissue characterisation of benign lesions (tumour and tumour-like) with the US is more specific than characterisation of malignant lesions.
- Calcified phleboliths in haemangiomas and matrix mineralisation in soft tissue tumours can be assessed.

Colour Doppler ultrasound is a non-invasive method for assessment of lesion vascularisation and blood vessel position. It helps in the assessment of the following parameters in the tumour under interrogation:

- Blood flow presence and intensity
- Pattern of vascularity (chaotic, Figure 2.1B, or organised)
- Tissue structure: solid and vascular part identification
- Vascular and lymphatic malformations have characteristic sonographic appearances.
- Haemangioma can be diagnosed without a need for biopsy.
- Doppler helps differentiate pseudoaneurysm from haematoma.

Pitfalls of the ultrasound:

- Lipoma variants, mechanical changes in benign lipomas and well-differentiated liposarcomas cannot be accurately differentiated.
- Haematoma cannot be differentiated from haemorrhagic solid soft tissue tumour (Figure 2.2).

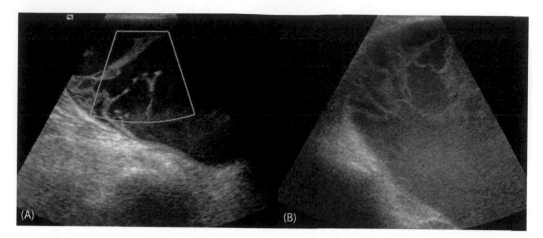

Figure 2.2: **Pitfalls of ultrasound: Ultrasound images show fairly similar appearances of large, predominantly cystic lesions with internal septations and internal foci. It is virtually impossible to differentiate Morel-Lavalle lesion overlying the left greater trochanter (A) from a completely haemorrhagic biopsy grade III sarcoma (B). (Image Courtesy of Dr. Harun Gupta.)**

- Fluid differentiation is not possible (infected versus non-infected).
- Differentiation of peripheral vascularity, whether due to pathological vessels or the compression of the normal adjacent small vessels, cannot be observed.

Advantages of US over MRI are lack of partial volume effect, short examination time and absence of motion artefacts. US limitations include the inability to show the deepest part of the deeply located lesions (depending on the probe) and cases with tumour extension adjacent to bone. During US-guided core needle biopsies, one should target vascularised areas and avoid areas of necrosis.

MRI should be performed when US fails to establish a specific diagnosis or when the margins of the lesion cannot be presented clearly (e.g. deep seated lesion, superficial fascia affection, size >5 cm and in suspicion of tumour recurrence after excision).

● *Radiography*

Radiography serves a limited role in the evaluation of soft tissue sarcomas. However, it may give information about calcifications and mineralisation, involvement of the adjacent bone (bony cortex destruction, presence and type), delineation of the soft tissue planes and mass density.

Chest radiography is the first-line examination and follow up since most soft tissue tumours metastasise the lungs.

- Calcification pattern analysis (osteoid, chondroid and dystrophic) within the soft tissue tumour may predict tissue type.
- Poorly defined amorphous calcifications may indicate synovial sarcoma and extraskeletal osteosarcoma in a large, aggressive soft tissue mass (Figure 2.3).
- Osteocartilagenous masses favour the diagnosis of synovial chondromatosis.
- Phleboliths – circular calcifications with lucent centres – suggest haemangioma (Figure 2.4A).
- Radiographs can aid in diagnosing some tumour mimics such as myositis ossificans (Figure 2.4B) and tumoral calcinosis (Figure 2.4D).

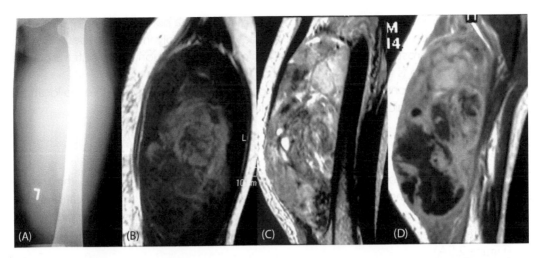

Figure 2.3: Radiography in aggressive soft tissue tumour: Anteroposterior radiograph
(A) through the left thigh shows a large soft tissue density shadow overlying the left
femur. There are no secondary bony changes or soft tissue calcifications seen. Synovial
sarcoma, sometimes, may demonstrate cortical erosions or amorphous calcification.
The large soft tissue lesion on radiograph proved to be high-grade synovial sarcoma on
T1-weighted (B), T2-weighted (C) and post-contrast T1-weighted non-fat-suppressed
(D) images.

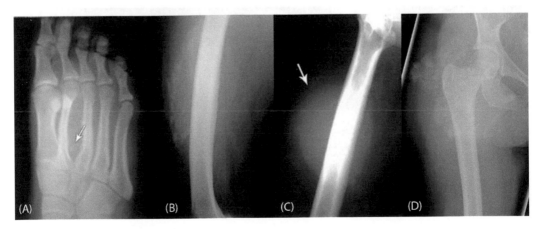

Figure 2.4: Various soft tissue pathologies on radiographs: Oblique dorsoplantar
radiograph (A) through the left foot shows a well-circumscribed calcification (arrow
marked) with internal radiolucent centre (phlebolith) characteristic of underlying
slow-flow vascular malformation. (B) Lateral radiograph through the right femur shows
well-formed calcification oriented along the vastus lateralis muscle fibres consistent
with myositis ossificans (please refer to Figure 2.5A for CT appearances). (C) Soft
tissue shadow on radiograph through the right femur in a different patient suggests
a large deep lesion (arrow marked) potentially involving thigh musculature, and
(D) anteroposterior radiograph through the right hip and proximal femur shows globules
of amorphous calcification around the right hemipelvis. Subsequently the patient has
had a CT and an MRI demonstrating tumoral calcinosis (please refer to Figure 2.5E for
CT appearances).

- Soft tissue tumours abutting the bony cortex may induce a bone reaction (Figure 2.4C), pressure erosion or bony invasion. The degree of bony involvement may be presented as cortical hyperostosis (parosteal lipoma) or cortical destruction at the outer aspect of the cortex which is termed as "saucerisation".
- Radiograph limitations are small lesions without mineralisation, masses with deep locations or complex anatomical areas such as the pelvis and spine.

● *Computed tomography*

The attenuation values of soft tissue sarcomas are slightly lower compared to the muscle density. The highest density comes from calcifications, mineralisation and ossifications. Pre-contrast CT is necessary for the differentiation of calcifications from vascular enhancement.

- Peripheral irregular and coarse calcification typically appear in myositis ossificans (Figure 2.5A).
- Fat tissue tumours with low density can be depicted with CT. However, the presence of dense nodular structures is in favour of low-grade liposarcomas.
- Tumoral margins are better appreciated following contrast application due to increased density of the vascularised tumour compared to the surrounding normal tissue. It is helpful for better demarcation of potentially necrotic areas.
- CT angiography is used to assess tumour viability and vascularity, vascular relationship and preoperative planning (Figure 2.5B).

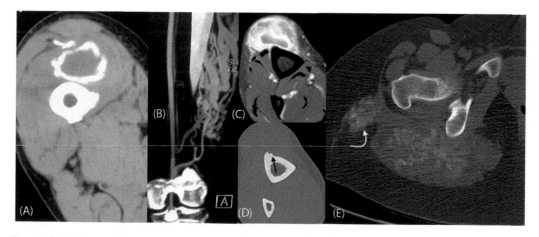

Figure 2.5: **Uses of computed tomography (CT): (A) Non-contrast axial CT image through the right femoral shaft shows peripherally calcified lesion with a thin rim of soft tissue between the native femur and the calcified mass consistent with myositis ossificans within the right vastus intermedius muscle. (B) MIP reformatted coronal CT image through the distal thigh demonstrates a large vascular malformation with feeding vessels from the popliteal artery. (C) Post-contrast T1-weighted fat-suppressed axial image shows aggressive necrotic soft tissue mass, biopsy proven synovial sarcoma, intimately related to the anteromedial surface of the tibial midshaft. (D) Underlying cortical erosion (black arrow) at the anteromedial tibial cortex is better seen on axial non-contrast CT image. (E) Non-contrast axial CT image in a bone window shows fluffy calcification in the musculature around the hip joint with layering of liquified calcium (curved arrow) consistent with tumoral calcinosis.**

- The relationship of the tumour with the adjacent bone is more accurately depicted with CT than with radiography, especially when the tumour is in complex anatomical regions. Extrinsic osseous cortex remodelling or invasion is more accurately detected (Figure 2.5C and D).
- Performing volume rendering allows better spatial orientation, which is more important for surgeons and closer to their perspective of lesion viewing in the operating room (Figure 2.5B).
- CT is used to biopsy soft tissue lesions within the deep and complex anatomical region.
- CT is used to detect lung metastases (without contrast) whereas pulmonary angiography detects pulmonary embolism (incidence of unsuspected pulmonary embolism is 1 to 5%).
- CT for local staging of primary malignant tumours should be performed in cases when MRI is contraindicated or in cases with metal implants (Figure 2.5E).

● *Magnetic resonance imaging*

MRI is the gold standard imaging technique for evaluating soft tissue sarcomas.

MRI can assess the location, size, intra- or extra-compartmental location, margins and presence of pseudocapsule, fascial relationship, peritumoral oedema, infiltration of adjacent structures, such as vessels, nerves, bones, joints, and the distance from the skin (Figure 2.6).

MRI can detect various tissue signal intensities (tissue morphology including fat, fluid and blood), homogeneity, vascularity, enhancement pattern, necrotic, haemorrhagic, fluid-fluid levels, cystic areas, presence of multiple lesions and enlarged lymph nodes (Figure 2.6).

Selection of appropriate FOV, imaging planes, MRI sequences and the necessity for contrast application is explained in subsequent text.

Field of view
- FOV is selected and adjusted according to the size and location of the mass. FOV must be large enough to study the entire lesion, including peritumoral oedema and the surrounding areas of normal tissue, to perform adequate local staging.
- A large FOV may result in loss of spatial resolution. However, it can be beneficial if multiple lesions are suspected in the given anatomical region or a comparison with the opposite side is needed.
- Limited large FOV is an option for occult soft tissue lesions requiring specific anatomical landmarks.

Imaging planes and slice thickness
- True axial plane must be taken through the entire lesion to better assess the neurovascular and compartmental relationship. At least one orthogonal plane to the axial images is also mandatory. It can be selected depending upon the anatomical location of the lesion. For instance, the sagittal plane can better demonstrate a lesion involving the anterior and posterior thigh soft tissue, whereas a coronal plane is recommended for the lesion involving medial and lateral soft tissues.
- Slice thickness should be a maximum of 4 mm or 3 mm in smaller lesions.

MRI sequences
No single imaging sequence is sufficient to provide all necessary information. One must use the MRI sequences in conjunction with each other to provide adequate information. At least

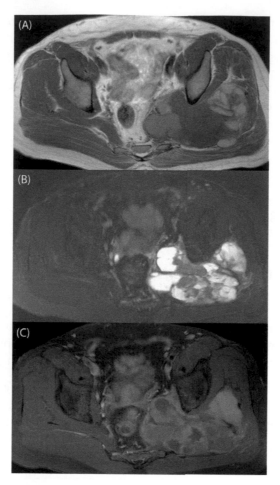

Figure 2.6: Magnetic resonance imaging (MRI) in soft tissue sarcoma: (A) T1-weighted, (B) STIR and (C) post-contrast T1-weighted fat-suppressed axial MRI images at the level of acetabular roof show a large aggressive lesion involving the left deep gluteal muscles and hemipelvis. The lesion shows soft tissue, cystic/necrotic, fatty and enhancing components. The MRI can demonstrate anatomical relationships, extension and neurovascular relations better than any other imaging modality. "Triple-signal" sign is seen on MRI and this was confirmed as synovial sarcoma on histopathology. (Image Courtesy of Dr. Harun Gupta.)

one T1-weighted and one fluid-sensitive sequence (such as T2 fat saturated or short-tau inversion recovery [STIR] sequence) should be used.

T1-weighted images

Soft tissue tumours are generally isointense to muscle and it is extremely difficult to demarcate them from the involving muscle. Conversely, the tumour is very well-demarcated when it is entirely within the subcutaneous layer due to the high soft tissue contrast of the surrounding fat.

- T1-weighted (T1W) images allow the demarcation of anatomical structures, neurovascular bundles and subcutaneous fat. Preservation of fat planes is essential for surgical planning due to clear tumour delineation by intermuscular and subcutaneous fat tissue (Figure 2.7A). Therefore, an axial T1W non-fat suppression is obligatory.

- T1W images improve the structural assessment of the tumour. The majority of soft tissue tumours have homogenous signal intensity. Internal high T1W signal intensity is usually from the fat (Figure 2.7C), methaemoglobin (Figure 2.7B), melanin or protein-aceous fluid. Fat can be confirmed on fat suppression in corresponding areas using fat-suppressed sequences.
- They help differentiate viable areas from cystic parts in some tumours (Figure 2.7C), which may dramatically change the surgical approach.
- Axial T1W image is the baseline for contrast-enhanced studies.

Fluid-sensitive sequences with fat suppression

These should be used to better present the inhomogeneous high signal intensity tumour tissue and the high signal intensity of perilesional oedema. Both should be included in the radiological report because those should be resected in the definitive operative treatment. Peritumoral oedema often contains satellite micronodules.

- **T2-weighted images with fat suppression** can be used to confirm fat content within the tumour and increase the delineation of non-lipomatous components in lipoma-tous tumours (differentiation of lipoma from well-differentiated liposarcoma, Figure 2.8).
- **STIR** gives uniform fat suppression but needs a longer scan time for better signal to noise ratio (SNR) than the chemical shift-based fat-suppressed technique, where acqui-sition time is shorter with better SNR, but the fat suppression is less uniform.

Fat-suppressed T1W images are not used commonly. They almost always used a pre-contrast imaging sequence for direct comparison with the post-contrast T1-FS sequence. We prefer non-contrast T1W to check post-gadolinium enhancement.

T2-weighted images are used for comparison of signal intensity to the muscle (low), fat (intermediate) and fluid (high), which is essential for tumour tissue characterisation. It may help differentiate myxoid lesions (demonstrate fluid signal intensity) and collagenous/fibrous lesions with low to intermediate signal intensity.

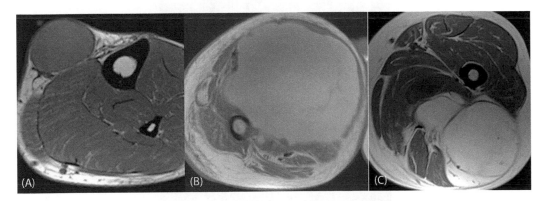

Figure 2.7: Various appearances on T1-weighted images: (A) Well-defined hypointense solid subcutaneous mass lesion (undifferentiated pleomorphic sarcoma) with a thin plane of preserve fat between the deep fascia anteromedially. (B) In a different patient, T1-weighted axial image through the midthigh shows a large hyperintense soft tissue mass consistent with haemorrhagic tumour – grade III sarcoma (please refer to Figure 2.2B for ultrasound images). (C) T1-weighted axial image in a well-differentiated liposarcoma shows mainly fatty signal and a small non-adipose component at the medial margin of lesion. (Image Courtesy of Dr. Harun Gupta.)

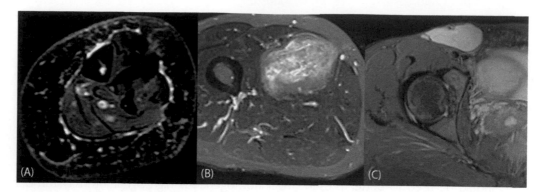

Figure 2.8: Various appearances on STIR images: Three different patients showing (A) simple forearm lipoma with complete fat suppression, (B) grade I liposarcoma in the midthigh with lack of fat suppression and oedematous changes, and (C) myxoid liposarcoma which has homogeneous high signal with complete lack of fatty signal on imaging.

Gradient-echo imaging (GRE) can be used in cases where haemangioma, mature haematoma, intratumoral haemorrhage or PVNS are suspected (Figure 2.9), it assesses the blood product deposition.

Contrast-enhanced MRI allows accurate local staging, better tumour margins delineation and tissue characterisation by improving demarcation of the viable tumour areas from

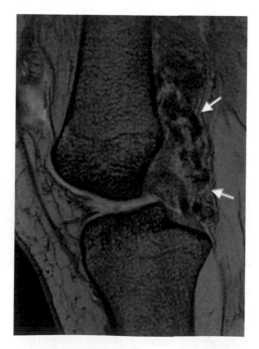

Figure 2.9: PVNS on a gradient-echo (GRE) image: Solid soft tissue within the posterior recesses of the knee demonstrates susceptibility artefacts also known as "blooming artefacts" on GRE image. The MRI appearances are characteristic of PVNS. (Image Courtesy of Dr. Harun Gupta.)

necrotic, cystic and myxoid areas in a solid tumour. In addition, tumoral haemorrhage and adjacent structural infiltration are diagnosed better by this technique.

- Surgeons prefer T1W imaging without fat suppression after Gadolinium administration because they have information about the fat planes and anatomical details, and the enhanced tumour is well presented. The main weakness is the lack of tumour-to-fat contrast.
- Malignant masses generally show a greater peak and rate of enhancement.
- Benign and malignant soft tissue tumours show overlapping enhancement patterns.
- Differentiating haematomas and haemorrhagic sarcomas is incredibly challenging. Sometimes, tumour nodules which are not visible on unenhanced sequences can be identified on post-contrast images.
- Subtraction imaging can be performed in patients with metal fixation.
- Solid and the most viable part of the tumour, depicted by intensely enhancing part, should be selected for imaging-guided biopsy planning.
- MR parameters on contrast-enhanced images in favour of malignancy are early dynamic enhancement (within 6 seconds after arterial enhancement), peripheral or inhomogeneous dynamic enhancement and rapid initial dynamic enhancement followed by a plateau or washout phase (please see Figure 14.3 in Chapter 14).

Diffusion-weighted imaging

Diffusion-weighted imaging (DWI) as functional imaging can be added to non-contrast MRI protocol. It is used for tumour detection, characterisation and treatment monitoring with qualitative and quantitative assessment. Highly cellular tissues with intact cell membrane and with small extracellular compartment have higher restrictions, presented with a high signal intensity of DWI (restricted diffusion) and low apparent diffusion coefficient (ADC) values (dark on ADC map).

- ADC values may give additional information in distinguishing benign from malignant lesions and in combination with standard MR parameters, may improve tumour characterisation. However, there are no universally applicable ADC values that may fit all lesions. Heterogeneity of malignant tumour tissue results in a variation of ADC values, which overlap with benign lesions.
- Higher-grade sarcomas have lower mean ADC values than well-differentiated sarcomas (please refer to Figure 14.1 in Chapter 14).
- Restricted diffusion helps identify small pelvic lymph nodes.
- DWI is useful in assessing treatment response after neoadjuvant chemotherapy.
- A potential pitfall of DWI may be the qualitative assessment of the tumour signal intensity. Tumours in DWI can have the same signal intensity as fluid in T2W imaging (T2 shine through). In such cases, qualitative findings should be correlated with ADC maps.

Chemical shift imaging

Chemical shift imaging is a technique based on gradient-echo imaging by cancelling out fat and water signals in a single voxel from similar quantities. It assesses the presence of microscopic fat within the lesion in percentage. Its application is limited to assessing the microscopic amount of fat in higher-grade liposarcomas (research application).

Whole-body MRI

There is a recommendation to use whole-body MRI for staging of myxoid liposarcomas as a small number of them can lead to skeletal metastasis which cannot be easily diagnosed on other imaging modalities such as CT or nuclear medicine bone scans. Similarly, whole-body

MRI remains the gold standard imaging technique for diagnosis and follow up of neurofibromatosis type I (please refer to Figure 5.5 in Chapter 5).

● MR spectroscopy

Proton MR spectroscopy represents a quantitative assessment technique for choline metabolite, a surrogate marker for cell membrane turnover, elevated in malignant soft tissue tumours. It is a time-consuming technique with most of the research value.

● Nuclear scans

Role of positron emission tomography (PET)-CT is established for work up of various malignancies; however, its role in routine assessment of soft tissue sarcomas is not yet defined. Certain sarcomas such as myxoid liposarcomas and synovial sarcomas demonstrate inherently low update and therefore the use of PET-CT is limited in these subtypes. Certain benign lesions such as hibernomas can demonstrate avid uptake (please refer to Figure 3.15 in Chapter 3). Therefore, PET-CT is best used as problem solving modality on case-by-case basis such as in patients with neurofibromatosis with malignant peripheral nerve sheath tumour (MPNST) (Figure 2.10).

Take-home points

● Suspected soft tissue sarcomas require a thoroughly investigative approach, including clinical history, prior imaging and relevant surgical suspicion narrowing the differential diagnosis.

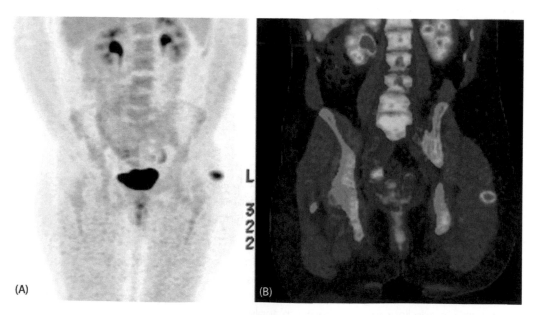

(A)   (B)

Figure 2.10: **Malignant peripheral nerve sheath tumour (MPNST) on PET-CT: 25-years-old patient with a medical history of neurofibromatosis type I presented withrapidly enlarging painful mass in the left buttock (biopsy proven MPNST) shows avid radiotracer uptake (A) within the lesion on PET-CT (B) performed to stage the lesion. (Image Courtesy of Dr. Harun Gupta.)**

- US is the first modality of choice for evaluation of soft tissue lesions that may give sufficient details about tissue structure, allowing differentiation of benign and tumour-like lesions from actual tumours in many cases.
- MRI is the gold standard imaging technique providing multiplanar imaging, excellent soft tissue contrast resolution and details about tumour spread, relationship, and locoregional assessment.
- CT gives additional information about the presence of calcifications and tumour matrix mineralisation in addition to other tumour components, and CT angiography plays an essential role in preoperative planning.

SUGGESTED READING

- Carra, BJ, Bui-Mansfield, LT, O'Brien, SD, Chen, DC. Sonography of musculoskeletal soft-tissue masses: Techniques, pearls, and pitfalls. AJR Am J Roentgenol. 2014 Jun;202(6):1281–1290.
- Fayad, LM, Jacobs, MA, Wang, X, Carrino, JA, Bluemke, DA. Musculoskeletal tumors: How to use anatomic, functional, and metabolic MR techniques. Radiology. 2012;265(2):340–356.
- Kransdorf, MJ, Murphey, MD. Imaging of soft-tissue musculoskeletal masses: Fundamental concepts. Radiographics. 2016 Oct;36(6):1931–1948.
- Noebauer-Huhmann, IM, Weber, MA, Lalam, RK, Trattnig, S, Bohndorf, K, Vanhoenacker, F, Tagliafico, A, van Rijswijk, C, Vilanova, JC, Afonso, PD, Breitenseher, M, Beggs, I, Robinson, P, de Jonge, MC, Krestan, C, Bloem, JL. Soft tissue tumors in adults: ESSR-approved guidelines for diagnostic imaging. Semin Musculoskelet Radiol. 2015 Dec;19(5):475–482.
- Vanhoenacker F, Parizel PM, Gielen J. Imaging of soft tissue tumors. Switzerland: Springer; 2017.

3 *Lipomatous tumours*

Siddharth Thaker, Harun Gupta

INTRODUCTION

Lipomatous tumours are one of the most common soft tissue lesions. They demonstrate a variety of imaging appearances and can be challenging to the radiologist when showing atypical appearances on ultrasound and/or magnetic resonance imaging (MRI). Sometimes, it is impossible to differentiate lipoma with secondary changes, such as fat necrosis, lipoma variants like spindle cell lipoma or hibernoma, or lipoma mimics such as soft tissue hae-mangioma and liposarcoma, based on imaging alone. When overlooked, liposarcoma can contribute to increasing patient morbidity and mortality. This chapter provides an overview of imaging appearances of lipomatous tumours with a predominant focus on ultrasound and MRI characteristics. It also underpins the need for multidisciplinary team involvement while managing lipomatous tumours with atypical features and outlines a sample referral strategy for radiologists or sonologists depending upon imaging features.

The latest World Health Organization (WHO) classification for soft tissue and bone tumours, published in 2020, has divided lipomatous tumours into an exhaustive list, seg-regated into three categories (Table 3.1): benign, intermediate (locally aggressive) and malignant. Immunohistochemistry, molecular genetics and histopathological characteristics risk-stratify the fatty tumours in the classification. Sarcomas are typically managed by a team consisting of radiologists, sarcoma pathologists, surgeons, sarcoma nurses and radiation

Table 3.1: **Lipomatous/Adipocytic Tumours (WHO classification 2020)**

Benign
Lipoma NOS (intramuscular lipoma, chondrolipoma)
Lipomatosis (diffuse lipomatous, multiple symmetrical lipomatosis, pelvic lipomatosis, steroid lipomatosis and HIV lipodystrophy)
Lipomatosis of nerve
Lipoblastoma and lipoblastomatosis
Angiolipoma NOS, myolipoma, chondroid lipoma
Spindle cell lipoma
Atypical spindle cell/pleomorphic lipomatous tumour
Hibernoma (tumour of mature brown fat)
Intermediate (locally aggressive)
Atypical lipomatous tumour
Malignant
Liposarcoma, well-differentiated (NOS, lipoma-like, inflammatory, sclerosing)
Dedifferentiated liposarcoma
Myxoid liposarcoma
Pleomorphic liposarcoma (epithelioid)
Myxoid pleomorphic liposarcoma

DOI: 10.1201/9781003218722-3

Table 3.2: Role of the Radiologist in the Management of Lipomatous Tumours

Stage of lipomatous mass evaluation	Role of radiologist
Presurgical stage	Perform imaging and establish lipomatous nature of the mass by excluding mimics, e.g. ganglion, vascular malformation and indeterminate soft tissue masses. Categorise lipomatous mass correctly into: • Non-aggressive lipoma requiring no further imaging • Lipomatous lesion with atypical features or potentially aggressive features and requiring multidisciplinary team (MDT) attention Review cases in the sarcoma MDT with discussion for: • Image-guided biopsy • Follow up or surgical removal depending upon patient and tumour factors
Post-surgical stage	Have routine postoperative follow-up imaging pathway Evaluate follow-up imaging, ascertain potential recurrence or metastasis

oncologists providing specific management-related inputs. The role of a radiologist is elaborated in Table 3.2.

Tasks for the radiologist presented with a fatty lesion involve answering the following questions:

• Is it a simple lipoma or not?
• If so, is it typical benign or atypical lipoma?
• Are there any concerning, indeterminate or aggressive features?
• Is biopsy and involvement of oncology and pathology needed?
• If removal is required, what vital structures may be compromised?

The radiologists must follow a rigorous imaging ritual to answer these questions and consider onwards referral based on their local and regional guidelines when needed.

IMAGING MODALITIES IN LIPOMATOUS LESIONS

● *Ultrasound*

• It is the initial imaging modality of choice for superficial palpable lesions.
• On ultrasound, assess for location (relation to deep fascia), size, echogenicity, septa and Doppler flow.
• If the lesion is sizable, a panoramic setting is recommended to cover the lesion completely. The authors encourage the panoramic or extended field view compared to the split images as the latter may not give the 'true' dimensions of the lesion (Figure 3.1).
• Use power Doppler to assess vascularity or disorganised flow. Linear septal flow is frequently seen in benign lesions and is considered normal. Similarly, peripheral capsular flow is also frequent and indicates compression of tiny vessels around the lesion rather than a true neovascularity. Disorganised intralesional flow is a concerning feature (Figure 3.2).
• Margins/capsule of the lesions located in the subcutaneous layer is sometimes seen better with ultrasound than MRI due to the higher resolution of ultrasound (Figure 3.3).

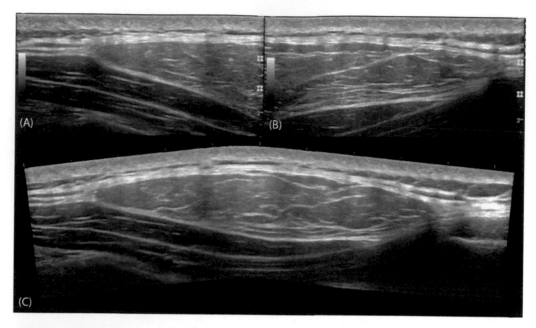

Figure 3.1: Importance of extended ultrasound view. Two contiguous greyscale ultrasound images (A) and (B) where the reader has to assume that the images are contiguous and represent the accurate dimension of the lesion. Please compare it to a panoramic image (C) showing the actual 'length' of the lesion.

The prime objective of the ultrasound is to differentiate the benign lipoma showing typical features from those with atypical features. The transition from the benign to malignant ultrasound features is further described later in the chapter under subheadings of intermediate and malignant lipomatous masses.

Depending upon ultrasound appearances, the radiologist can recommend (1) no further imaging if the lesion shows benign characteristics (described later in the chapter) or (2) MRI with or without a need for biopsy should there be any deviation from the benign ultrasound features. Ultrasound is also a modality of choice where image-guided biopsy is required.

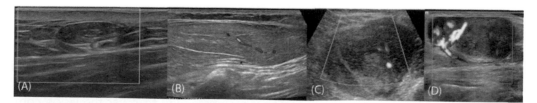

Figure 3.2: Patterns of vascularity in lipomatous lesions. Colour Doppler images in four different lipomatous lesions show various vascularity patterns. (A) A small vessel in the periphery of a fatty lesion represents a compressed vessel, and (B) a small vascular channel passing through a fine vascular septum – a common feature of a benign lipoma. Compare it with the images of (C) well-differentiated and (D) dedifferentiated liposarcomas from two different patients where it shows disorganised intralesional vascularity. Vascularity becomes more disorganised as the lesion becomes more dedifferentiated and aggressive.

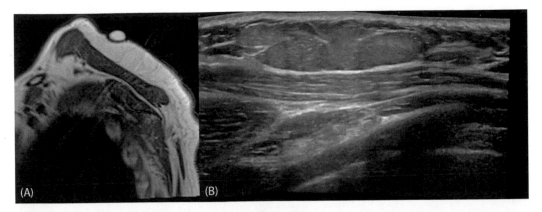

Figure 3.3: Utility of ultrasound in detecting superficial lipomatous lesions. T1-weighted sagittal image through the posterior upper neck (**A**) shows no apparent soft tissue lesion in a patient presenting with a lump at the marker site. (**B**) High-resolution greyscale ultrasound in the same patient showed a well-capsulated superficial lipomatous lesion. Ultrasound can detect and characterise superficial lipomatous tumours much better in many instances than MRI, given its higher spatial resolution for superficial structures.

● *Magnetic resonance imaging*

- MRI is considered a problem-solving modality for fatty lesions not showing the typical benign ultrasound features.
- It is the modality of choice for deep-seated and/or larger lesions where internal signal and anatomical characterisation are complex (Figure 3.4).
- Recommended MRI sequences are T1-weighted and a fat-saturated sequence such as T2-FS or short-tau inversion recovery (STIR); performed in two planes, with at least one of them being an axial plane. We do not recommend routine use of MRI contrast to assess these lesions.
- Benign lipoma, especially with secondary changes such as pressure-related MR signal changes, and atypical lipomatous tumours/well-differentiated liposarcoma, show overlapping MRI characteristics. Therefore, a further biopsy may be considered as histopathology and cytogenetics may be needed for the definitive diagnosis (Figure 3.5).

As a general rule, a lesion loses its typical fatty signal characteristic as its malignant potential increases. Thus, more fat equates to a lower grade of malignancy, higher-grade liposarcomas usually show minimal or virtually no fat.

- In presurgical planning, MRI provides critical information about the neurovascular bundles traversing near the potentially aggressive fatty lesion. Whole-body MRI is used in myxoid liposarcoma to detect any systemic bony metastatic involvement.
- In the post-surgical period, MRI is critical in detecting local complications, including recurrence.

● *Computed tomography scan*

- CT scan can evaluate the lipomatous lesions when MRI is contraindicated (Figure 3.6).
- It is useful in the detection of fatty lesions adjacent to/or within the bone (Figure 3.7 – periosteal lipoma)

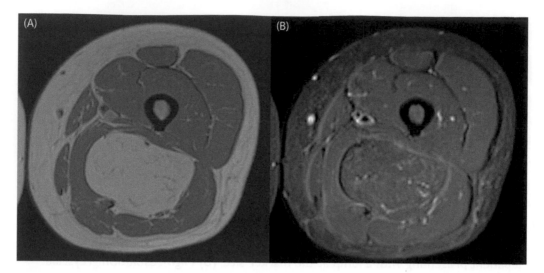

Figure 3.4: Use of MRI in the characterisation of deep lipomatous lesions. T1-weighted (A) and STIR (B) images of a large deep lipomatous lesion showing numerous fine septae and inhomogeneous fat suppression. However, it is challenging to differentiate lipoma variants and atypical lipomatous tumours with such imaging appearances. Hence, we performed an ultrasound-guided biopsy. Final diagnosis: hibernoma. In addition, MRI can help triage lesions into those requiring no further imaging or follow up or biopsy.

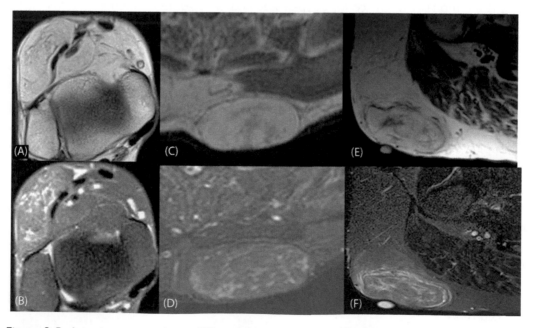

Figure 3.5: Imaging conundrum. T1-weighted (A) and STIR (B) images in a benign lipoma at the ankle with pressure-related changes. T1-weighted (C) and STIR (D) images of biopsy-proven spindle cell lipoma; T1-weighted (E) and STIR (F) images of a biopsy-proven atypical lipomatous tumour with *MDM2* gene amplification. All lesions show overlapping MRI features, namely, heterogeneous (non-fatty) internal signals on T1-weight images and inhomogeneous fat suppression on STIR.

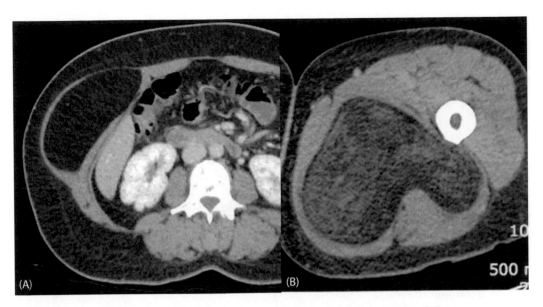

Figure 3.6: Use of CT in lipomatous lesions. Contrast-enhanced axial CT image (A) showing well-defined intramuscular lipoma within the right external oblique muscle without aggressive features. Compare it to image (B) at the level of the proximal thigh in a different patient showing internal heterogenous radiodensity suggesting an atypical lipomatous tumour. Histological diagnosis: dedifferentiated liposarcoma.

- CT is the gold standard imaging technique to detect and follow up on well-differentiated liposarcoma in the retroperitoneum, mediastinum and scrotum (Figure 3.8).
- Staging CT chest is used in higher-grade liposarcomas for assessing for lung metastases (see later in malignant lipomatous neoplasm).

We will discuss the imaging appearances of lipomatous masses according to WHO classification for easier understanding.

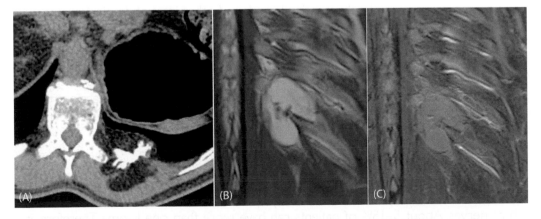

Figure 3.7: Periosteal lipoma. Axial CT image (A) in a patient with left lower rib mass showing a lipomatous lesion intimately related to the native rib with serpiginous calcified channels within it consistent with periosteal response to it and T1-weighted (B) and STIR (C) coronal images through the same lesion showing benign imaging appearances.

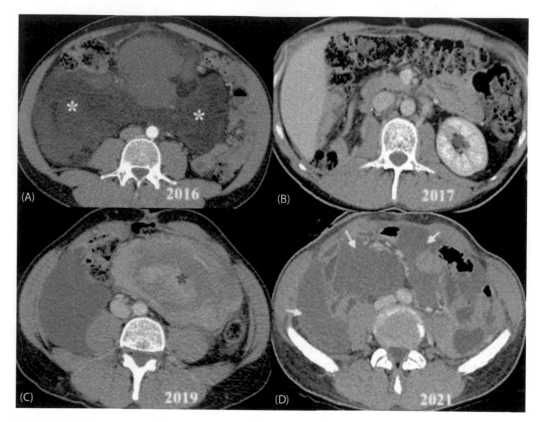

Figure 3.8: CT to detect and follow retroperitoneal liposarcoma. (A) Contrast-enhanced CT shows a large multicompartmental fat density lesion (white asterisks) filling the entire retroperitoneal space. (B) Immediate follow-up with CT shows no residual tumour. (C) The patient presented with abdominal distension when CT showed recurrent, relatively solid appearing lesion in the retroperitoneal compartment on the left (red asterisk) consistent with tumour recurrence. It was resected along with multiorgan resection to achieve maximum tumour load reduction, and (D) follow-up CT showing diffuse re-recurrence completely encasing bowels and other intra-abdominal organs.

BENIGN LIPOMATOUS MASSES

Weiss and Goldblum have classified benign lipomatous masses into five categories – lipoma, lipoma variants, lipomatous tumours, infiltrating lipomas and hibernoma – again predominantly based upon cellular and anatomical characteristics.

● *Typical lipoma*

Typical lipoma is a benign, painless, slow-growing lesion that can occur virtually anywhere in the body. However, it may sometimes cause symptoms due to the mass effect on structures such as nerves. About 5–15% of patients can have more than one lipoma. Therefore, it is worth asking the patient if they have any other similar lesions when scanning them.

Ultrasound features

The typical ultrasound features of a benign lipoma include homogeneous mass, no or septal linear power Doppler flow and no or thin septa of less than 2 mm (Figure 3.9). Therefore,

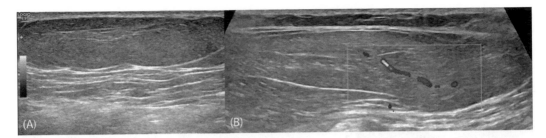

Figure 3.9: Benign superficial lipoma. Greyscale (A) and colour Doppler (B) ultrasound images showing ultrasound features of a classic benign lipomatous lesion. Please note the superficial location, fine septations, lack of internal non-fatty areas on greyscale imaging and septal vascular flow on the Doppler image.

ultrasound is usually diagnostic when typical appearances are present and superficial, and immediate subfascial lipomas do not need further imaging with MRI in cases when they can be covered entirely by ultrasound imaging.

MRI features

Typical benign lipoma demonstrates a homogenous bright signal, similar to the subcutaneous fat in the same image, on T1-weighted images, which shows complete and homogenous fat suppression in fat-suppressed images (Figure 3.10). Lipoma can involve any anatomical site (Figure 3.11). Therefore, it is helpful to comment on muscle fibres traversing through the lipoma when it is deep-seated. Such lesions are challenging to excise en masse (Figure 3.12).

Sometimes, benign lipoma demonstrates areas of inhomogeneity due to pressure effects or fat necrosis and can be challenging to differentiate from aggressive lesions. It is wise to perform a biopsy following a multidisciplinary team discussion in such cases.

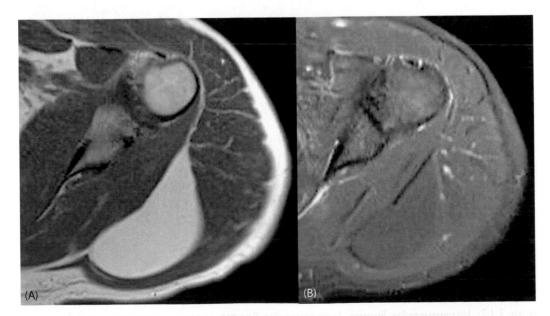

Figure 3.10: MRI features of benign lipoma. T1-weighted (A) and STIR (B) MRI images in a patient with a left shoulder intermuscular completely lipomatous lesion showing homogenous fat suppression on STIR images and benign imaging appearances.

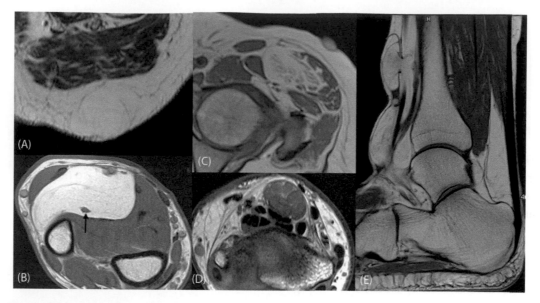

Figure 3.11: Locations of lipomatous lesions. Lipomatous tumours can involve any anatomical site in the body. They can be superficial (A), deep – appreciate deep forearm lipoma surrounding the ulnar nerve – black arrow (B), intramuscular (C), involving the nerve – lipomatosis of the median nerve (D) and intratendinous – showing extrusion into the subcutaneous fat through defects (curved red arrow) within the tendon sheath (E).

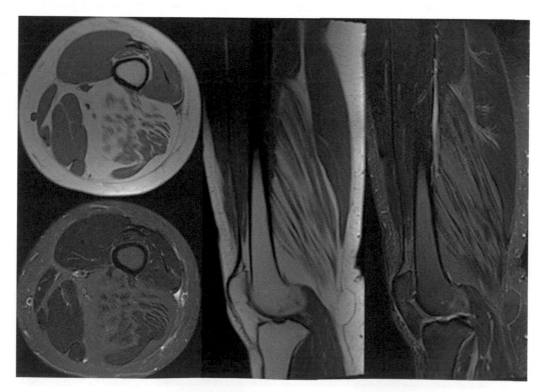

Figure 3.12: Intramuscular lipoma. Intramuscular lipoma contains numerous muscle fibres (biceps femoris) through the lesion. It is an important finding to mention in the reports. These can mimic non-adipose areas on imaging and make it difficult to resect the lipomatous lesion en masse needing consent for potential loss of muscle and function.

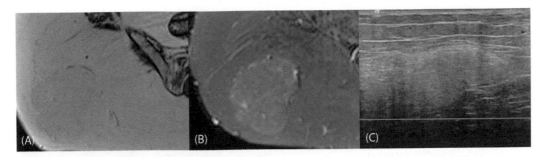

Figure 3.13: Hibernoma. T1-weighted (A) and STIR (B) images in a patient with a right buttock mass showing a large subcutaneous lesion with inhomogeneous fat signal intensity and corresponding STIR signal heterogeneity. On greyscale ultrasound (C), the lesion appears predominantly fatty with shadowing areas and an ill-defined inferior border.

● *Lipoma variants*

These are benign lipomatous lesions such as spindle cell lipoma, angiolipoma, hibernomas and pleomorphic lipomas (see Table 3.2). Typically, these are painless lesions apart from angiolipomas which may be painful.

Imaging features

These lesions are predominantly fatty but characterized by inhomogeneous fat suppression and sometimes internal vascularity on imaging.

On ultrasound, this can be in the form of non-homogeneous echogenicity and the presence of increased Doppler flow. On MRI, apart from the fat signal, there can be a variable degree of inhomogeneity on T1-weighted and STIR or T2 fat-suppressed images (Figure 3.13).

The different subtypes show considerable overlap in imaging and it is impossible to provide a definitive diagnosis based on imaging alone. For example, a well-encapsulated, subcutaneous fatty lesion in the posterior neck showing heterogenous appearances on MRI and thin septa on ultrasound which shows intense septal enhancement on post-gadolinium, increases the possibility of spindle cell lipoma as the final diagnosis (Figure 3.14). Lipoma variants such as angiolipoma and hibernoma may show increased radiotracer uptake (appearing hot) on PET-CT and mimic malignancy (Figure 3.15).

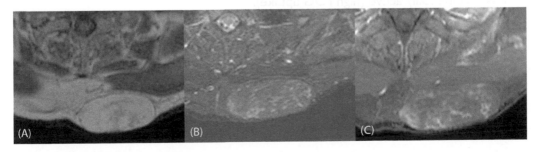

Figure 3.14: Spindle cell lipoma. Typical appearances of the spindle cell lipoma in the posterior thoracic wall subcutaneous tissue. T1-weighted (A) and STIR (B) images show an inhomogeneous fatty lesion with thick internal septae, which show intense septal enhancement in the post-gadolinium image (C).

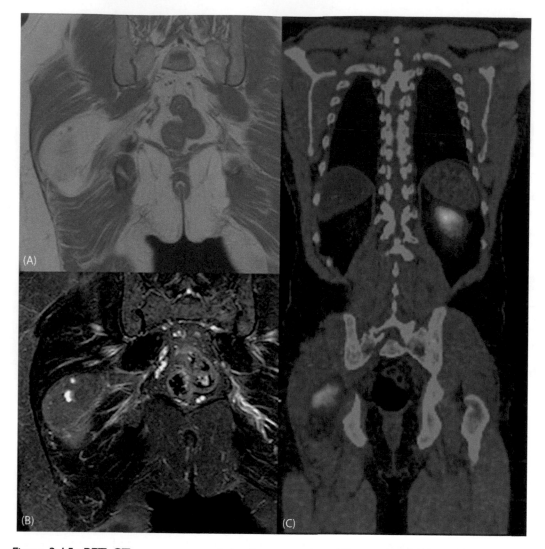

Figure 3.15: PET-CT appearances of the lipoma variant. T1-weighted (A) and STIR (B) images in a patient with a deep lipomatous lesion involving the right gluteus maximus with internal areas of cystic degeneration/necrosis showing increased radiotracer uptake on PET-CT (C). The lesion was proven to be hibernoma (tumour containing brown fat) which is metabolically active (high FDG uptake).

INTERMEDIATE LIPOMATOUS MASSES

According to the latest WHO classification, these include atypical lipomatous tumours (ALT). The terminology is reserved for lipomatous masses in extremities that show *MDM2* gene amplification regardless of the aforementioned 'typical' or 'atypical' imaging features and can be wholly excised when required. In addition, they do not have metastatic potential but tend to recur locally.

● *Ultrasound features*

ALT should be suspected on ultrasound when presented with fatty mass showing concerning ultrasound features such as nodular areas of non-fat signal in a deep lipomatous mass

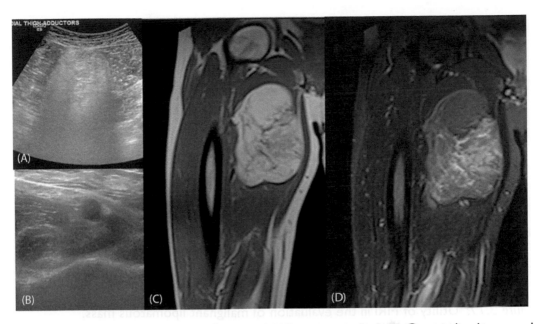

Figure 3.16: Imaging appearances of an atypical lipomatous tumour. Greyscale ultrasound image (A) showing a large deep lipomatous mass within the right adductor compartment with intense posterior acoustic shadowing and (B) echo poor non-fatty areas within it. A subsequent MRI was performed, given the highly suspicious nature of the lesion. T1-weighted (C) and STIR (D) images showed thick irregular septations, non-fatty soft tissue areas (not shown) and excessive signal heterogeneity. Histopathological diagnosis: grade I liposarcoma.

(Figure 3.16). Other aggressive features include disorganised vascularity, blurred margins, low-fat proportion and encasement of neurovascular structures.

● MRI features

These lesions show heterogeneous signals on T1-weighted and incomplete fat suppression on STIR images. In addition, they can produce a significant mass effect on surrounding structure, involve multiple muscles of the same compartment, displace or uncommonly encase neurovascular bundles and show extra compartmental extension (Figure 3.17).

● Lipoma variant v/s atypical lipomatous tumour

The imaging features of lipoma variant and ALT show considerable overlap, and it is often impossible to differentiate one from the other based on imaging alone. We have described salient features of lipoma variants and ALT in Table 3.3. There is a small risk of dedifferentiation in ALT cases (approximately 6%) to a higher-grade liposarcoma.

Lipomas and lipoma variants do not undergo malignant transformation. Therefore, sometimes when there is a lack of clarity in imaging diagnosis, it is worth doing a biopsy for a conclusive diagnosis. If required, these can be managed conservatively.

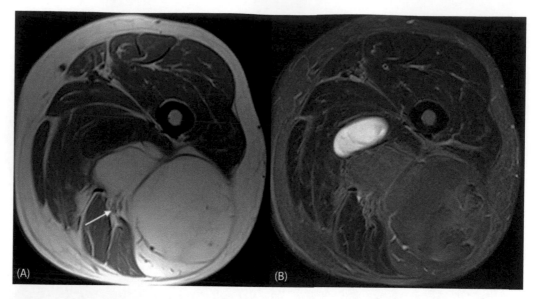

Figure 3.17: Utility of MRI in the evaluation of malignant lipomatous mass. T1-weighted (A) and STIR (B) images in a biopsy-proven atypical lipomatous tumour/well-differentiated liposarcoma showing multicompartmental involvement (medial and posterior compartments are involved) and close relationship with the sciatic neurovascular bundle (white arrow). There is a large non-adipose area in the anterior medial aspect of the lesion.

MALIGNANT LIPOMATOUS MASSES

The term "well-differentiated liposarcoma" is reserved for locally aggressive lipomatous masses having characteristics similar to ALT in extremities but involving mediastinum, retroperitoneum or scrotum, where even with multiorgan resection, complete tumour excision is not possible. The latest WHO classification includes dedifferentiated, myxoid, pleomorphic and myxoid pleomorphic liposarcomas in the malignant lipomatous masses categories. These types are based upon the lesion's cellular makeup, including myxoid and round cell components, besides the fatty content and *MDM2* gene amplification.

Table 3.3: Salient Features and Differences between Lipoma Variants and atypical lipomatous tumours

	Lipoma variant	ALT
Grade	Benign	Intermediate
Imaging features	Variable but typically inhomogeneous fat suppression	Variable but typically inhomogeneous fat suppression
Clinically concerning features		Age > 60 years, lower limb, deep-seated
Typical fat content	Majority fat	Majority fat
MDM2	Negative	Positive
Metastatic potential	No	No
Recurrence	Locally	Locally
Dedifferentiation to higher grade	No	Yes Approximately in 6% cases

As per the general rule, the lesion loses its typical fatty imaging characteristic as its malignant potential increases. Thus, more fat equates to a lower grade of malignancy; higher-grade liposarcomas usually show minimal or virtually no fat on imaging.

● *Ultrasound features*

One should suspect aggressive lipomatous lesion when ultrasound features are concerning, such as minimal fat, heterogeneous appearances, invasive margins and disorganised power Doppler flow (Figure 3.18). Therefore, MRI is usually recommended for such lesions.

● *MRI features*

As mentioned before, the fat content of the lipomatous lesion decreases as its malignant potential increases. In malignant masses, the fat may virtually be absent or present in the minimal amount on MRI. MRI provides an excellent overview of the lesion's size, extent and architecture including cystic, myxoid and necrotic components; involvement of neurovascular bundles, joints and muscles; and detects locoregional metastatic spread.

Myxoid liposarcoma may show characteristic rounded myxoid areas within a deeply located fatty tumour (Figure 3.19).

Dedifferentiated liposarcoma shows virtually no fat and it is extremely challenging to differentiate it from other sarcomatous lesions (Figure 3.20). Both myxoid and dedifferentiated liposarcomas have high malignant potential. However, while dedifferentiated liposarcoma involves the lungs during metastatic spread, myxoid liposarcoma can rarely cause bone metastases (Figure 3.21).

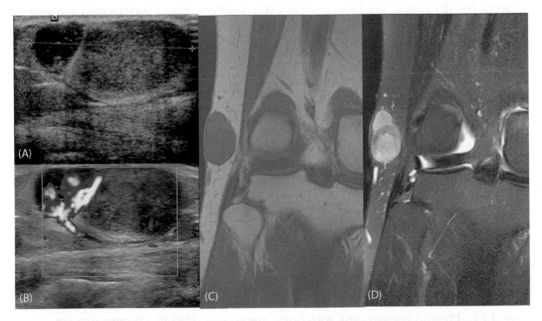

Figure 3.18: Dedifferentiated liposarcoma. Greyscale (A) and colour Doppler (B) images showing a non-fatty solid mass lesion with aggressive internal vascularity and corresponding T1-weighted (C) and STIR (D) images demonstrate a complete lack of fatty component in a differentiated liposarcoma within the lateral subcutaneous fat around the knee.

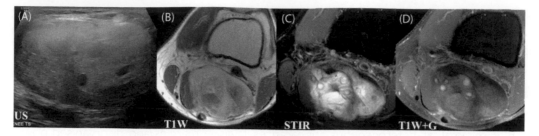

Figure 3.19: Myxoid liposarcoma. A subset of liposarcoma showing characteristic yet aggressive appearances on ultrasound (A) showing circular myxoid areas interspersed with fatty components and on MRI showing extensive myxoid matrix intermixed with fatty components on T1-weighted (B) and STIR (C) images. More intense enhancement of circular areas suggests solid myxoid nature (D) than cystic degeneration or fat necrosis.

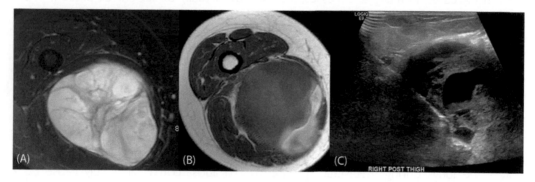

Figure 3.20: Dedifferentiated liposarcoma – a diagnostic challenge. T1-weighted (A) and STIR (B) images in a biopsy-proven (C) dedifferentiated liposarcoma showing complete absence of fat on MRI and ultrasound (C). In such cases, liposarcoma cannot be differentiated from other soft tissue sarcomas based on imaging alone.

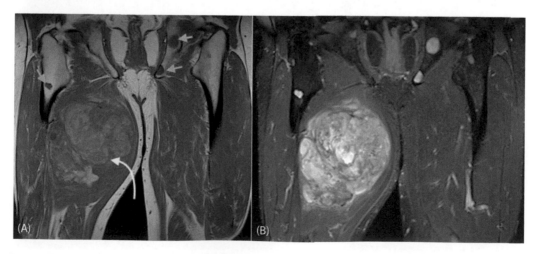

Figure 3.21: Myxoid liposarcoma with bony metastases. MRI in a biopsy-proven myxoid liposarcoma involving the right adductor musculature (curved yellow arrow) showing a large deep-seated aggressive mass lesion with solid soft tissue and internal haemorrhagic/necrotic areas on T1-weight (A) and STIR (B) images. Please note well-defined metastatic deposits within the right proximal femur and left ischium (amber arrows).

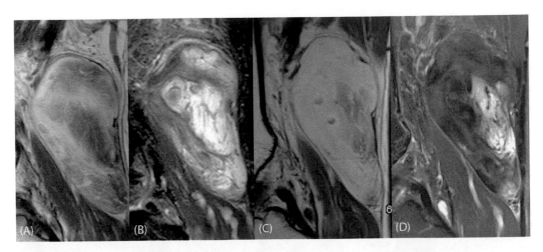

Figure 3.22: Neoadjuvant radiotherapy-related changes in myxoid liposarcoma. Therapy-related changes in a biopsy-proven myxoid liposarcoma tethered to the posterior knee capsule. Respective T1-weighted and STIR images before (A and B) and after (C and D) neoadjuvant chemotherapy showed a marked decrease in the myxoid component and increase in the fatty part, which was concordantly reflected on the excision sample on histopathology.

The MRI is also helpful in detecting neoadjuvant therapy-related changes (Figure 3.22) and recurrence following surgical excision (Figure 3.23).

Take-home points

- WHO classification categorises lipomatous lesions as benign, intermediate (ALT) and malignant.
- The radiologist's role is to segregate "benign lipoma with typical imaging features" from "lipomatous mass with non-typical imaging appearances".
- Ultrasound is sufficient for typical superficial lesions. Use an extended field of view to visualise longer lesions. It can show margins of superficial lesions better as compared to MRI. Linear Doppler flow is considered normal.
- MRI is useful for large, deep-seated lesions where detailed internal and anatomical characterisation is required.
- Typical lipoma diagnosis is straightforward on imaging.
- Lipoma variant versus ALT: It is difficulty to differentiate lipoma with mechanical changes, i.e. lipoma variants from ALT based on imaging alone. ALT behaves like a lipoma but has a small risk of dedifferentiation to higher-grade liposarcoma. Therefore, these often need biopsy and histopathological and cytogenetic analysis for diagnosis.
- Liposarcomas: Higher-grade liposarcomas typically have limited or no identifiable fat on imaging. A biopsy is required for their diagnosis.
- Follow-up cross-sectional imaging should be tailored according to the lipomatous mass's final histological type and grade.

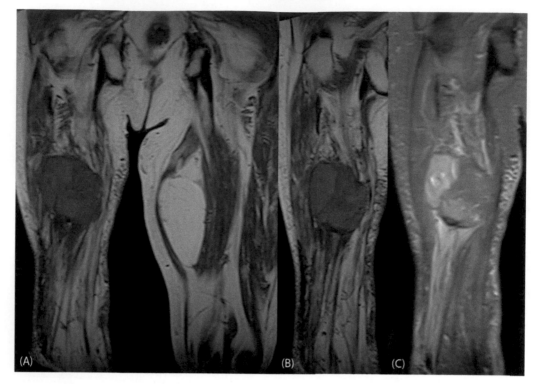

Figure 3.23: Recurrent and now dedifferentiated liposarcoma. Recurrent right thigh mass lesion in an 85-year-old male with a history of lump excision from the same site many years back and another lump in the left proximal thigh. T1-weighted image (A) showing non-fatty mass lesion (dedifferentiated liposarcoma) in the right thigh and intramuscular fatty mass lesion (biopsy-proven lipoma) in the left thigh. Cropped T1-weighted (B) and STIR (C) images show a complete absence of fatty components in the dedifferentiated lesion, and there are adjoining changes from previous treatment (post-surgical and post-radiotherapy changes).

SUGGESTED READING

- Brisson, M, Kashima, T, Delaney, D, Tirabosco, R, Clarke, A, Cro, S, Flanagan, AM, O'Donnell, P. MRI characteristics of lipoma and atypical lipomatous tumor/well-differentiated liposarcoma: Retrospective comparison with histology and MDM2 gene amplification. Skeletal Radiol. 2013 May;42(5):635–647.
- DeSchepper AM, Parizel PM, Ramon F, DeBeuckeleer L, Vandevenne JE, editors. Imaging of soft tissue tumors. New York: Springer Science & Business Media; 2013 Mar 9.
- Inampudi, P, Jacobson, JA, Fessell, DP, Carlos, RC, Patel, SV, Delaney-Sathy, LO, van Holsbeeck, MT. Soft-tissue lipomas: Accuracy of sonography in diagnosis with pathologic correlation. Radiology. 2004 Dec;233(3):763–767.
- Kransdorf, MJ, Murphey, MD. Imaging of soft tissue tumors. Lippincott Williams & Wilkins; 2006.
- WHO Classification of Tumours Editorial Board. Soft tissue and bone tumours. Lyon (France): International Agency for Research on Cancer; 2020. (WHO classification of tumours series, 5th ed. Vol. 3). https://publications. iarc.fr/588 (Last accessed on 11 September 2021)

4 Fibroblastic, myofibroblastic and fibrohistiocytic tumours

Ankit A Tandon, Jordan ZT Sim

INTRODUCTION

Fibroblastic, myofibroblastic and fibrohistiocytic soft-tissue tumours encompass a broad spectrum of mesenchymal tumours that are commonly encountered during clinical practice. The World Health Organization (WHO) classification (updated in 2020) of fibroblastic, myofibroblastic and fibrohistiocytic tumours categorised these tumours into benign, intermediate (locally aggressive and rarely metastasising) and malignant tumours (Tables 4.1 and 4.2).

The clinical manifestations of these tumours are widely varied, often with overlapping radiological and histopathological features. Although the imaging characteristics of these tumours may be non-specific, certain clinical features, in conjunction with the radiological findings, can shorten the list of differentials. This chapter provides an overview of imaging appearances of fibroblastic, myofibroblastic and fibrohistiocytic tumours, outlines a practical approach and offers insight into some of the most common lesions in each category. Important imaging and clinical features that can aid the radiologist in making an accurate diagnosis are emphasised (Table 4.3).

APPROACH TO IMAGING FIBROBLASTIC, MYOFIBROBLASTIC AND FIBROHISTIOCYTIC TUMOURS

Imaging characterisation of fibrous tumours should not be limited to magnetic resonance imaging (MRI). Each imaging modality has strengths and weaknesses and some can highlight certain features of a lesion better than others.

● Plain radiographs and computed tomography

- Help to distinguish hard palpable lumps caused by underlying bony deformity (e.g. exostosis).
- Best to assess soft tissue calcifications, e.g. myositis ossificans (Figure 4.1).
- Bony erosions and periosteal reactions are best seen on X-rays/computed tomography (CT) scans.
- CT is also frequently used to evaluate lesions located in the head and neck, mediastinum, chest wall (Figure 4.2) and retroperitoneum.

DOI: 10.1201/9781003218722-4

Table 4.1: **Fibroblastic/Myofibroblastic Tumours (WHO Classification 2020)**

Benign
Nodular fasciitis
Proliferative fasciitis and proliferative myositis
Myositis ossificans and fibro-osseous pseudotumour of digits
Ischaemic fasciitis
Elastofibroma
Fibrous hamartoma of infancy
Fibromatosis colli
Juvenile hyaline fibromatosis
Inclusion body fibromatosis
Fibroma of tendon sheath
Collagenous fibroma (desmoplastic fibroblastoma)
Myofibroblastoma
Mammary-type myofibroblastoma
Calcifying aponeurotic fibroma
EWSR1-SMAD3-positive fibroblastic tumour (emerging)
Angiomyofibroblastoma
Cellular angiofibroma
Angiofibroma NOS
Nuchal fibroma
Acral fibromyxoma
Gardner fibroma
Intermediate (locally aggressive)
Palmar/plantar-type fibromatosis
Desmoid-type fibromatosis
Lipofibromatosis
Giant cell fibroblastoma
Dermatofibrosarcoma protuberans
Intermediate (rarely metastasising)
Dermatofibrosarcoma protuberans, fibrosarcomatous transformation
Solitary fibrous tumour
Inflammatory myofibroblastic tumour
Low-grade myofibroblastic sarcoma
Superficial CD34-positive fibroblastic tumour
Myxoinflammatory fibroblastic sarcoma
Infantile fibrosarcoma
Malignant
Solitary fibrous tumour, malignant
Fibrosarcoma NOS
Myxofibrosarcoma
Low-grade fibromyxoid sarcoma
Sclerosing epithelioid fibrosarcoma

Abbreviation: NOS, not otherwise specified.

Table 4.2: So-called Fibrohistiocytic Tumours (WHO Classification 2020)

Benign
Tenosynovial giant cell tumour
Deep benign fibrous histiocytoma
Intermediate (rarely metastasising)
Plexiform fibrohistiocytic tumour
Giant cell tumour of soft parts NOS
Malignant
Malignant tenosynovial giant cell tumour

Table 4.3: Salient Features of Common Fibrous, Myofibroblastic and Fibrohistiocytic Tumours

Tumour	Typical patient age and gender	Typical tumour location	Important points
Nodular fasciitis	Younger patients (20–40 years)	Upper extremities (most common), trunk, head and neck, lower extremities	Inverted target sign, fascial tail sign Rapid growth can be confused with soft tissue sarcomas Known to spontaneously regress
Myositis ossificans	Young active males	Thigh	History of trauma, high T2 signal intensity (SI) in the early and subacute stages, gradual ossification in centripetal fashion; latter better appreciated on radiograph/CT scan
Elastofibroma dorsi	Women older than 55 years	Between posterior chest wall and inferior tip of scapula, deep to the latissimus dorsi and rhomboid major muscles Commonly bilateral	Fat entrapped within a soft lesion isointense to skeletal muscles in classic location in a middle-aged patient is pathognomonic
Fibroma of tendon sheath (FTS)	M:F = 2:1, middle aged patients	Wrist and hand Rare in feet	Closely related to tendon sheath No blooming on gradient
Collagenous fibroma (desmoplastic fibroblastoma)	50–70 years old men	Arm, shoulder, lower limb and back	Low to very low T1/T2 SI Rim enhancement is characteristic
Giant cell tumour of tendon sheath (GCTTS)	Third to fifth decade of life Slight female preponderance	Hands and feet	Low-intermediate T1 and T2 SI Blooming on gradient Thrice as common as FTS

(Continued)

Table 4.3: Salient Features of Common Fibrous, Myofibroblastic and Fibrohistiocytic Tumours (*Continued*)

Tumour	Typical patient age and gender	Typical tumour location	Important points
Palmar fibromatosis and plantar fibromatosis	Male, middle-aged patients	Palmar aponeurosis. Extension parallel to flexor tendons of fingers Medial band of plantar aponeurosis	Fascial tail sign Association with diabetes, epilepsy or alcoholism
Extra-abdominal desmoid tumours	Female, 25–40 years old	upper extremity, chest wall and thigh Can be multifocal	Extension into surrounding muscles and fascia Low T2 signal band-like structures representing collagenous content may help to d/d from soft tissue sarcomas
Solitary fibrous tumour	No gender predilection Middle-aged adults	Thoracic cavity, thigh and pelvic retroperitoneum	Large, solid vascular tumour with prominent perilesional vessels Paraneoplastic hypoglycaemia
Dermatofibrosarcoma protuberans	20–50 years old patients	Trunk (most common), extremities, head and neck	Unmineralised, nodular mass involving skin and subcutaneous tissues Claw sign at lesion–skin interface Fibrosarcoma variant – more aggressive form
Fibrosarcoma NOS (adult-type)	30–60 years old patients	Deep soft tissues of lower extremities	Heterogeneous, ill-defined, infiltrative mass Spoke-wheel pattern of enhancement Band-like areas of low SI suggestive of fibrous origin Usually occurs in relation to deep fascia
Myxofibrosarcoma	Fifth to sixth decade of life. One of the most common soft tissue sarcomas in elderly patients	Dermal and subcutaneous tissues	Infiltration along fascial planes as well in the deeper soft tissues Myxoid component: T1 hypo-, T2 bright which enhances relatively less compared to non-myxoid component of tumour

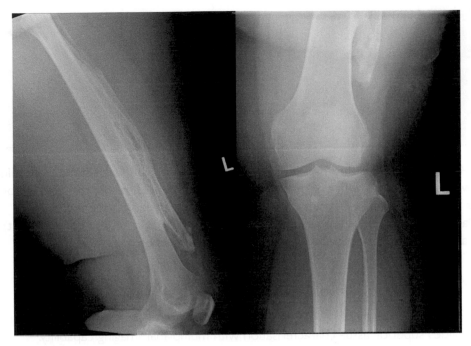

Figure 4.1: Plain radiographs of the left thigh and knee demonstrate heterotopic ossification almost along the entire length of the femur, forming sheet-like appearance (mature myositis ossificans). Lesions like myositis ossificans are easily followed up with radiographs, without the need for invasive biopsies or surgical intervention.

● *Ultrasound*

- Sonography is the initial imaging modality of choice for superficial palpable lesions.
- It is useful in differentiating solid from cystic lesions and determining size, internal morphology and vascularity of masses (Figure 4.3).
- Ultrasound is also used for image-guided percutaneous biopsies (Figure 4.5B(d)).

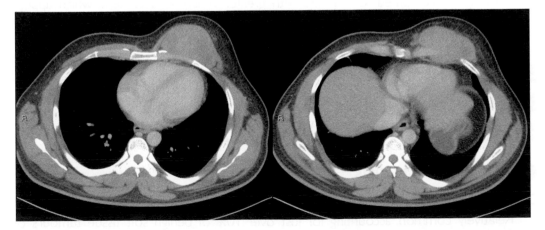

Figure 4.2: Computed tomography is an excellent modality for lesions in the chest and mediastinum. This example demonstrates a desmoid-type fibromatosis originating deep to the pectoralis muscle with involvement of the chest wall.

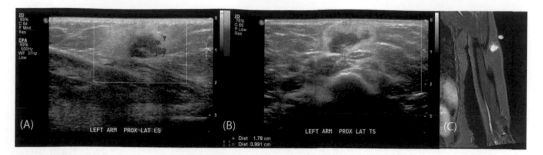

Figure 4.3: Ultrasound is the imaging modality of choice for superficial lesions. This middle-aged woman presented with a palpable lesion in her left arm. Ultrasound images in both planes (A and B) show an ill-defined lesion with thick hyperechoic walls and internal vascularity. The mass enhances avidly with contrast (C: T1 fat-saturated post-contrast) and was shown to be a dermatofibrosarcoma protuberans post resection.

● *Magnetic resonance imaging*

- MRI remains the mainstay for imaging soft tissue including fibrous tumours since it provides superior tissue characterisation with multiplanar imaging capability.
- It plays a key role in tissue characterisation of soft tissue tumours; determining their anatomical extent and relationship to adjacent structures; guiding surgical planning and post-treatment surveillance.
- Essential sequences to include in a fibrous tumour protocol are T1-weighted (T1W) (elastofibroma shows fatty streaks within), T2-weighted (T2W, hypointense collagenous bands) spin-echo sequences with fat saturation, short-tau inversion time recovery (STIR) sequence, gradient-echo sequences (fibrohistiocytic tumours show blooming due to hemosiderin) and, in some cases, post-contrast T1W fat-suppressed sequences in at least two orthogonal planes.
- Skin markers are useful to localise the post-operative scars and ensure that the palpable lump/region of interest has been included within the field of view (Figure 4.4).
- In general, cellular tumours tend to possess higher T2 signal and post-contrast enhancement when compared to tumours with greater collagenous content, which appear darker on T2 with more delayed contrast enhancement (Figure 4.9). Fibrous tumours characteristically are of hypointense to intermediate signal intensity on T2W images.

BENIGN FIBROBLASTIC, MYOFIBROBLASTIC AND FIBROHISTIOCYTIC TUMOURS

● *Nodular fasciitis*

Demographics

- Relatively common, accounting for just over 10% of benign soft tissue tumours of fibrous origin.
- Affects younger patients (mean age: 20–40 years).
- Affects men and women equally.

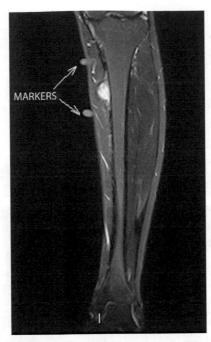

Figure 4.4: Skin markers. Coronal STIR image of a patient's calf with skin markers demarcating the region of interest. Skin markers are useful for radiographers to ensure the lesion in question is included in the field of view. They can also help to pinpoint the symptomatic lesion, especially if there are other lesions elsewhere in the study.

Aetiology
- May be due to a reactive process triggered by local injury or inflammation.
- A study by Mayo Clinic demonstrates association with the *MYH9-USP6* gene and thus suggests an underlying neoplastic nature.

Location and clinical features
- Typically located in the upper extremities (46%), trunk (20%), head and neck (18%) and lower extremities (16%).
- There are three subtypes based on lesion location: subcutaneous, fascial and intramuscular.
- Patients typically complain of a fast-growing palpable mass that may or may not be tender.

Imaging
- Ultrasound: Lesions typically appear hypoechoic and are sometimes seen with cystic change (Figure 4.5B(d)).
- CT: Usually demonstrates low attenuation due to its myxoid nature.
- MRI: Most of these appear with isointense to slightly hyperintense signal intensity to muscle on T1W images and heterogeneously hyperintense on T2W images. Figure 4.5A and B demonstrates the following features:
  - An "inverted target sign" is often seen; a central area of T2 hyperintensity with the low signal intensity seen in the periphery. The peripheral zone will show marked post-contrast enhancement with a poor enhancement of the central region.
  - A "fascial tail" characterised as thickening and enhancement of adjacent fascia is commonly seen with these lesions (Figure 4.5A(d)).

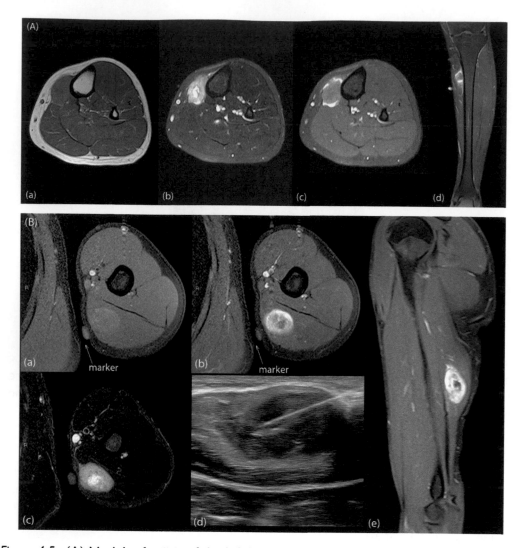

Figure 4.5: (A) Nodular fasciitis of the left leg in a 42-year-old male. (a–d) T1 pre-, T2, T1 post-contrast in axial and coronal planes demonstrate a soft tissue shin lesion with characteristic appearance of nodular fasciitis. An "inverted target sign" is seen with marked peripheral enhancement and relatively poorer enhancement of the central region. Note is also made of "fascial tail sign" on coronal post-contrast images. (B) Intramuscular nodular fasciitis, left upper arm in a young boy. A peripherally enhancing (T1 iso to hyperintense in a, T1 post-contrast in b and e) lesion is seen in the left triceps muscle. The characteristic "inverted target sign" is again demonstrated. Ultrasound-guided biopsy image (d) demonstrates an intramuscular, well-defined, hypoechoic solid lesion. The lesion spontaneously regressed on follow-up MRI study.

Management

- Rapid growth and non-specific MR appearance of nodular fasciitis may be confused for soft tissue sarcoma. Young age of patient may be clue to its diagnosis.
- Nodular fasciitis lesions may also spontaneously regress and hence histological correlation may enable a non-operative approach.
- If warranted, complete local excision is usually curative with recurrence seen in less than 2% of cases.

● *Myositis ossificans*

Demographics
- A self-limiting benign ossifying process that tends to occur in young active males.
- When it occurs in the periosteum of the digits, it is known as fibro-osseous pseudotumour of the digits; this particular entity occurs more commonly in young women.

Aetiology
- A history of trauma is reported in up to half of the cases.
- It can also occur with infection, coagulopathy, burns etc.

Location and clinical features
- Typically located in the proximal and anterior muscle groups, with the quadriceps femoris being the most commonly affected muscle.
- Tender soft tissue swelling that may become firm and hard after 2 to 3 weeks.

Imaging
- X-ray/CT: Ectopic ossification is often visible between 4 and 6 weeks after the initial trauma.
  - Changes will be seen in the form of lamellar bone formation starting at the periphery and advancing towards the radiolucent centre in a centripetal fashion (Figure 4.6A).
- Ultrasound: Depends on the stage and degree of calcification within the lesion, evolving from a heterogeneous hypoechoic mass into a highly reflective mass with an irregular calcified rim at maturation.
- MRI: Also depends on the stage of lesion maturation.
  - Early/acute stage: High T2 signal due to muscle necrosis and haemorrhage, often with a hypointense rim that enhances with contrast.
  - Intermediate/subacute stage (Figure 4.6B): T1 is iso- to hyperintense, T2 is hyperintense with a rim of the signal void representing calcification.
  - Mature/chronic stage: Signal voids corresponding to ossification become more extensive, often in an "onion-skin" pattern better appreciated on radiographs/CT.

Management
- Myositis ossificans is usually self-limiting. Follow-up radiographs may help avoid unnecessary biopsy and surgical intervention.

● *Elastofibroma dorsi*

Demographics and aetiology
- Generally seen in women older than 55 years.
- Thought to be secondary to repeated mechanical friction.

Location
- Occurs almost exclusively between the posterior chest wall and inferior tip of the scapula, deep to the latissimus dorsi and rhomboid major muscles, in close relation to the serratus anterior and ribs.
- Bilateral lesions are common and seen in up to 60% of patients.
- Patients may experience mild discomfort or restricted motion when moving the shoulder.

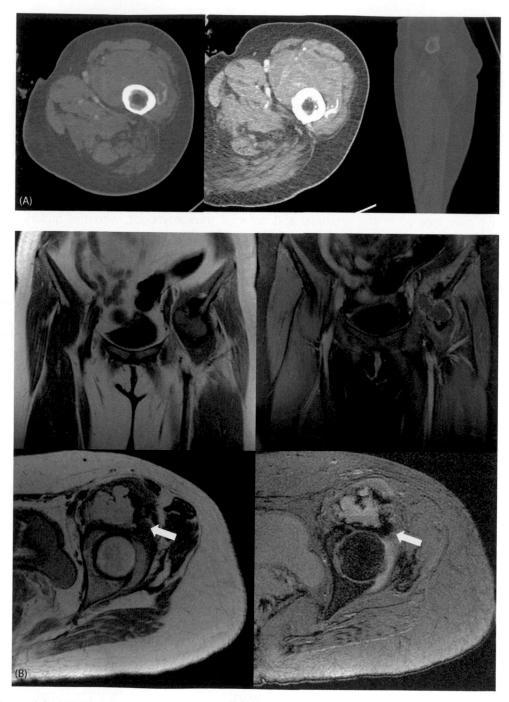

Figure 4.6: (A) Myositis ossificans, left thigh. Axial and sagittal reconstructed CT slices reveal a large haematoma in the muscles of anterior compartment of thigh mainly in the vastus intermedius and vastus medialis. Peripheral calcification is developing in the lateral margin of vastus intermedius haematoma. (B) Another patient of myositis ossificans, left hip. T1 pre- and post-contrast coronal, T2 and gradient echo axial images show myositis ossificans in subacute stage. Note the T1 and T2 hyperintense signal of the rim enhancing fluid collection along with layering compatible with hematoma formation. The collection is associated with developing rim of calcification blooming on gradient sequence. There was extensive oedema in the surrounding muscles as well from recent injury.

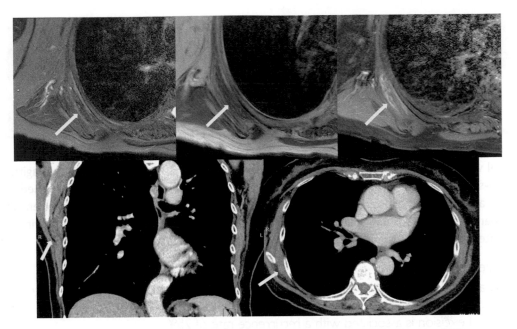

Figure 4.7: Elastofibroma dorsi. Axial T1, T2 fat-saturated and post-contrast MR images along with axial CT slices and coronal reconstruction demonstrate the typical appearance of elastofibroma dorsi (isointense to skeletal muscles with streaks of fat seen on MRI) at typical location between the posterior chest wall and inferior tip of the scapula, deep to the latissimus dorsi, in close relation to the serratus anterior and ribs.

Imaging (Figure 4.7)
- CT: Similar attenuation to muscle, sometimes with foci of low density similar to fat at characteristic location **(refer to arrows in** Figure 4.7 **CT images)**.
- MRI: Well-defined heterogeneous lentiform soft tissue mass with signal intensity like or slightly less than that of skeletal muscles.
  - Interlaced fatty tissues within the mass will show signal intensity similar to that of fat.
  - Finding of fat entrapped within a fibrous mass in a classic location in a middle-aged patient is pathognomonic of elastofibroma.

Management
- Surgery should be reserved for symptomatic patients. Local excision is curative.

● *Fibroma of tendon sheath*

Demographics and location
- Presents as a slow-growing mass in middle-aged patients.
- Twice as common in men as in women.
- Most commonly seen in the wrist and hand.

Imaging (Figure 4.8)
- Radiographs may demonstrate scalloping of the adjacent bone.
- MRI: Focal nodular mass closely related to the tendon sheath with low to isointense T1 signal, low to intermediate T2 signal with variable enhancement.
- Main differential on MRI is the giant cell tumour of the tendon sheath (GCTTS). Unlike GCTTS, FTS does not show blooming on gradient sequence.

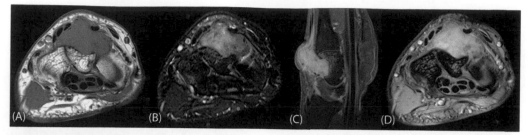

Figure 4.8: Fibroma of tendon sheath in a 53-year-old male patient presenting with stable dorsal wrist bossing over 5–6-month period. Axial T1 (A), T2 fat-saturated (B) and sagittal T1 fat-saturated post-contrast (C) images reveal a lobulated T1 isointense, T2 intermediate signal, avidly enhancing lesion in relation to extensor carpi radialis brevis and 4th extensor compartment tendons and splaying them. The lesion also causes scalloping of underlying capitate bone. GRE image (D) demonstrates no blooming artefact.

Management

- Diagnosis is made on histology which shows spindled fibroblasts within the collagenous stroma and characteristic slit-like vasculature.
- Local excision is associated with a recurrence rate of 25%.

● *Collagenous fibroma (desmoplastic fibroblastoma)*

Demographics and location

- Generally seen in men in their fifth and sixth decades of life.
- Common locations are the arm, shoulder, lower limb and back.
- Often involves the subcutaneous tissue, skeletal muscle and fascia.

Imaging

- MRI: Low to very low signal intensity on T1W/T2W images representing a predominantly collagenous matrix of these lesions (Figure 4.9).
- Characteristic rim enhancement is often seen due to outer capsule-like fibrous tissue with rich capillary covering.
- Appearance can be confused with desmoid tumours although collagenous fibromas are less cellular and infiltrative. Rim enhancement is also a useful differentiating factor.

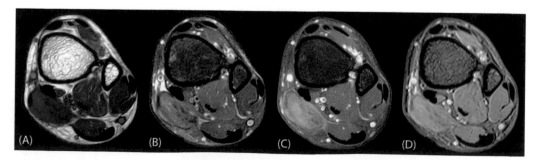

Figure 4.9: Collagenous fibroma close to medial malleolus in a 50-year-old male patient. Axial T1 (A) and T2 fat-saturated (B) images reveal a fairly well-marginated T1 iso- to hypointense, T2 intermediate to hypointense lesion in the subcutaneous tissues abutting the flexor tendons. On post-contrast images (C), the lesion demonstrates heterogeneously internal enhancement along with the characteristic rim enhancement of capsule. GRE image (D) demonstrates no blooming artefact.

Management
- Definitive treatment is marginal excision; accurate pre-operative diagnosis is imperative to prevent overtreatment.

● *Giant cell tumour of tendon sheath or tenosynovial giant cell tumour*

Demographics and location
- Typically affects patients in third to fifth decade of life.
- A predilection for hands and feet.

Imaging (Figure 4.10A)
- GCTTS represents a focal extra-articular form of pigmented villonodular synovitis (PVNS; Figure 4.10B – intra-articular PVNS) and thus possesses similar imaging features.
- MRI: Low to intermediate signal intensity on T1W/T2W sequences due to collagenous stroma with blooming artefact on gradient sequences; generally show strong post-contrast enhancement.
- X-ray: May demonstrate pressure erosion of adjacent bone. Internal calcifications are extremely uncommon and other diagnoses, such as fibro-osseous pseudotumour when it occurs in digits, should be considered, especially in young women.
- Ultrasound: Homogeneous hypoechoic mass with internal vascularity that does not move with flexion or extension of the tendons.
- Main differential is fibroma of tendon sheath (FTS); GCTTS is almost three times as common, and FTS is extremely rare in the feet.

Management
- Local excision is the treatment mainstay although recurrence is seen in up to 44% of cases.

INTERMEDIATE LOCALLY AGGRESSIVE FIBROBLASTIC AND MYOFIBROBLASTIC TUMOURS

● *Fibromatosis (superficial and deep)*

Fibromatoses cover a wide range of benign fibroblastic proliferation (Table 4.4). Enzinger and Weiss classified them into superficial (fascial) and deep (musculoaponeurotic) types and further subcategorised them according to anatomical location.

Superficial fibromatosis
Palmar fibromatosis or Dupuytren's contracture (Figure 4.11A)
- Presents as nodular or band-like soft tissue masses arising from proximal palmar aponeurosis and extending along with subcutaneous tissues of the finger in parallel to flexor tendons. Eventually, a cord-like structure forms, resulting in flexion contracture of the affected finger.
- Associated with diabetes, epilepsy and ethanol-induced liver disease.

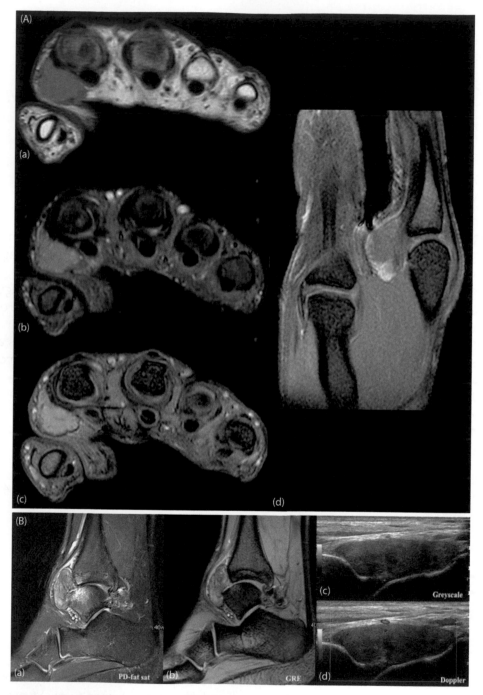

Figure 4.10: (A) Tenosynovial giant cell tumour in the hand in a 33-year-old female. A longitudinally oriented T1 and T2 (a, b) intermediate to hypointense signal intensity mass closely related to flexor tendon sheath of second finger with peripheral blooming on gradient sequence (c). It shows eccentric enhancement on post-contrast images (d). (B) Intra-articular tenosynovial giant cell tumour/PVNS of the ankle. (a) T2 fat-suppressed and (b) gradient echo (GRE) sagittal images of the right ankle showing a solid hypointense mass with areas of signal-dropout on GRE images involving the anterior ankle joint with reactive marrow oedema due to chronic mechanical changes in the anterior talus and tibial plafond. Corresponding greyscale (c) and Doppler (d) ultrasound images show a solid mass lesion without internal disorganised vascularity.

Table 4.4: Superficial and Deep Fibromatosis

Superficial (fascial) fibromatosis	Palmar fibromatosis (Dupuytren's contracture) Plantar fibromatosis (Ledderhose's disease) Penile fibromatosis (Peyronie's disease) Knuckle pads
Deep (musculoaponeurotic) fibromatosis	Extra-abdominal fibromatosis Abdominal fibromatosis Intra-abdominal fibromatosis • Pelvic fibromatosis • Mesenteric fibromatosis • Gardner's syndrome

- It is by far more frequent in men and can be seen in patients with a family history.
- MRI: Low signal intensity on T1W/T2W sequences with "fascial tail sign"; linear extension of lesion along aponeurosis, seen best after contrast administration.
- These tend to recur when excised in their cellular phase.

Plantar fibromatosis or Ledderhose's disease (Figure 4.11B)

- Affects men in their fourth decade of life.
- Associated with epilepsy, alcoholism and neuropathy.
- Usually involves the non-weight bearing medial band of the plantar aponeurosis.
- Ultrasound: Appears as a hypoechoic nodule superficial to the plantar aponeurosis.
- MRI: Low to intermediate signal intensity on T1W/T2W sequences depending on pre-dominance of collagenous or cellular content. Arises from deep plantar aponeurosis and typically blends with underlying plantar musculature.
- Often treated conservatively with footwear modifications; surgical resection can see recurrence rates of 40%.

Deep fibromatosis: Extra-abdominal desmoid tumours

- These are larger and generally show more aggressive behaviour than superficial fibromatoses.
- Peak incidence is between 25 and 40 years of age with a predominance in women of childbearing age.
- Extra-abdominal desmoid tumours are associated with familial adenomatous polyposis.
- These can occur anywhere in the body, although most commonly seen in the upper extremity, chest wall and in thighs. Can be multifocal (Figure 4.12A – fascial and deep fibromatoses involving the leg and fascial fibromatosis in the foot in the same patient).
- These never metastasise but multicentric, synchronous and metachronous presentations have been reported.
- Infiltration into the surrounding muscles and fascia is frequent and bony involvement is seen in up to 37% of cases. Locally aggressive lesions can be confused with soft tissue sarcomas.
- Ultrasound: Show variable echogenicity and can demonstrate marked shadowing as a result of a large amount of dense collagen within the mass (Figure 4.12B(a)).
- MRI: Can appear lobulated, irregular or stellate. (Figure 4.12B(b, c))
  - Early stage cellular lesions demonstrate T2 hyperintensity while mature collagenous lesions tend to show low signal intensity on T1W/T2W sequences.

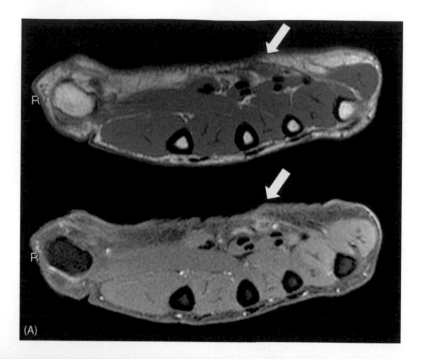

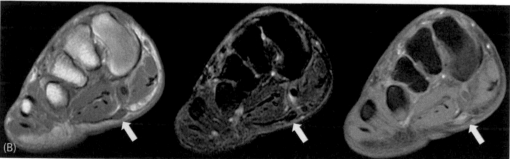

Figure 4.11: (A) Palmar fibromatosis or Dupuytren's contracture in the left hand in a 57-year-old male. T1-weighted pre- and post-contrast (above and below respectively) axial images of the left hand show a subcutaneous nodule over the palmar surface of the ring finger (arrows). The linear extensions of the lesion along the aponeurosis are best seen in the post-contrast images. (B) Plantar fibroma in a 45-year-old male. T1 iso- to hypointense, T2 hypointense, mildly enhancing plantar fibroma is seen arising from the medial cord of plantar aponeurosis.

- Low signal band-like morphology due to collagenous bands can help clinch the diagnosis (Figure 4.12B **arrows**) when trying to differentiate from soft tissue sarcomas.
- "Fascial tail sign" can also be seen with fascial involvement (Figure 4.12A(a, b) **curved arrow**).
- Treatment is wide surgical excision, although recurrence rates average around 40% due to its infiltrative nature. Radiofrequency ablation can be an alternative treatment when surgery is less feasible.

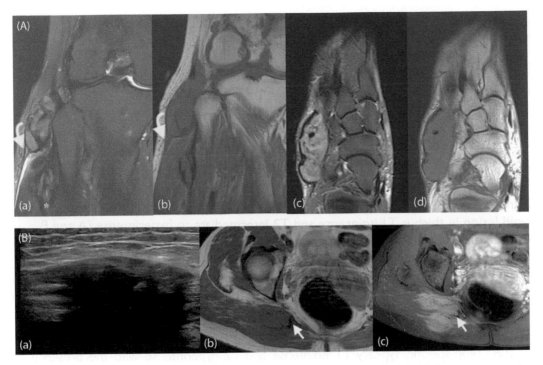

Figure 4.12: (A) Multifocal fibromatoses in leg, knee and foot. Sagittal T2 fat-suppressed (a) and T1-weighted non-contrast (b) images demonstrate T1 isointense, T2 hypointense masses involving the deep fascia of the leg with tail sign (curved arrow) and the lateral compartment muscles of the leg (asterisk). Similar T2 fat-suppressed (c) and T1-weighted (d) characteristics lesion is also seen arising from the deep fascia around the ankle/ hindfoot laterally. (B) Ultrasound and MRI features of the deep fibromatosis. Greyscale ultrasound image (a) showing a solid mass lesion with dense acoustic shadowing consistent with fibrous nature of the lesion. MRI demonstrates T1-weighted (b) isointense and T2 fat-suppressed (c) hyperintense lesion involving the right gluteus maximus muscle. Low-signal band-like morphology (arrows) can help clinch the diagnosis.

INTERMEDIATE RARELY METASTASISING FIBROBLASTIC AND MYOFIBROBLASTIC TUMOURS

● *Solitary fibrous tumours*

Demographics and location:

- Solitary fibrous tumours (SFTs) are most often seen in middle-aged adults with no predilection for either gender.
- These can occur anywhere in the body but are most commonly seen in the thoracic cavity, thighs and pelvic retroperitoneum.
- Large SFTs can cause paraneoplastic hypoglycaemia by producing insulin-like growth factors.
- Malignant lesions are often larger than 10 cm, demonstrating infiltration and heterogeneous appearance on imaging.

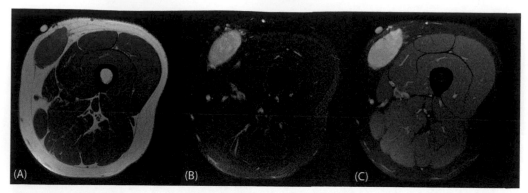

Figure 4.13: Solitary fibrous tumour in the left thigh of a 32-year-old male. Superficial, ovoid lesion in thigh is T1 isointense and T2 intermediate to hyperintense (A and B, respectively) with marked contrast enhancement (C). Prominent perilesional vessels are also noted. Imaging features may be confused with dermatofibrosarcoma protuberans especially when located in the subcutaneous tissues; histological correlation is usually warranted.

Imaging features (Figure 4.13)
- MRI: Non-specific, typically T1 isointense and T2 hyperintense with the presence of prominent perilesional vessels and marked enhancement.
- Diagnosis is made on histology which shows the characteristic branching haemangiopericytoma-like vessels and positive staining with CD34.

Management
- Surgical removal is often curative in benign lesions while prognosis is variable in more malignant tumours. One study showed a 70% 10-year survival rate.

● *Dermatofibrosarcoma protuberans*

Demographics and location
- It is the most common cutaneous sarcoma and accounts for approximately 6% of all soft tissue sarcomas.
- Patients' age tends to be between 20 and 50 years.
- Trunk is the most common site of occurrence followed by extremities and head and neck region.
- Since it is a slow-growing lesion, patients tend to present late.

Imaging features (Figure 4.14A and B)
- Ultrasound: Well-defined, lobulated lesion with echogenic foci and posterior acoustic enhancement and peripheral vascularity (Figure 4.3).
- CT: Unmineralized, nodular, homogeneously enhancing mass involving the skin and subcutaneous tissue. Larger lesions may show internal areas of necrosis and cystic degeneration.
- MRI: Most features are non-specific:
  - Well-defined lesion that is isointense on T1W and intermediate to hyperintense on T2W sequence. It shows intermediate to marked enhancement on post-contrast sequence.
  - "Claw sign" at the lesion–skin interface due to tentacle-like projections from the tumour is seen in most cases (Figure 4.14A and B).

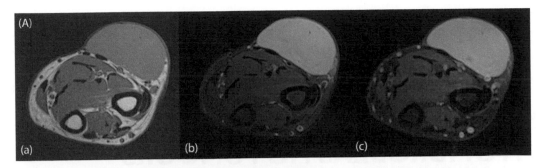

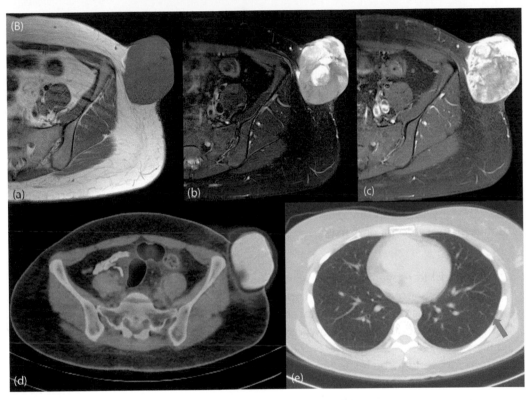

Figure 4.14: (A) Dermatofibrosarcoma protuberans (DFSP) in a 42-year-old male patient. A large, well-marginated homogeneously slightly T1 hyperintense (a), T2 bright (b) lesion showing avid enhancement on post-contrast images (c) is demonstrated in the subcutaneous tissues of the forearm. Note the appendages arising from the tumour surface. (B) Dermatofibrosarcoma protuberans (DFSP) with fibrosarcomatous transformation in a 33-year-old female patient. A large, exophytically growing T1 iso- to slightly hyperintense (a), T2 heterogenous intermediate to high signal intensity (b) lesion, showing heterogeneous but avid enhancement on post-contrast images (c), is demonstrated in the skin and subcutaneous tissues of the left side of trunk. Note the appendages arising from the tumour surface. Lesion also shows avid FDG uptake on PET CT study (d). Follow-up chest CT demonstrates a small pulmonary metastasis in the left lower lobe (e). Based on these two cases, T2 heterogeneity within DFSP may warrant exclusion of fibrosarcomatous transformation.

Management
- Generally excellent prognosis after complete resection but tends to recur if inadequate surgical margins obtained. Fibrosarcoma variant (classified under intermediate rarely metastasising category) has a higher tendency for local recurrence and distant metastasis which is most often to lungs. Imatinib is effective as chemotherapeutic agent for the latter.

MALIGNANT FIBROBLASTIC AND MYOFIBROBLASTIC TUMOURS

● *Fibrosarcoma NOS (not otherwise specified)*

Demographics and location
- Two types exist: infantile and adult; the infantile-type fibrosarcoma is histologically identical to the adult-type but carries a much more favourable prognosis and is thus classified under intermediate rarely metastasising tumour while the adult-type is considered highly malignant.
- Occurrence peaks between 30 and 60 years of age.
- It predominantly occurs in the deep soft tissues of the trunk, and upper and lower extremities.
- The aetiology of adult fibrosarcoma remains unclear with associations seen with radiation therapy, as secondary differentiation in a solitary fibrous tumour, within dedifferentiated liposarcoma or it may even present as a cutaneous fibrous sarcoma.

Imaging features
- Ultrasound: Heterogeneous mass with ill-defined margins and internal vascularity.
- MRI: Heterogeneous mass with T1 hypo- to isointense signal and T2 low intermediate to hyperintense signal, with the enhancement of the tumour periphery in a spoke-wheel-like pattern. Band-like areas of low signal intensity within the tumour on T1W and T2W images are generally suggestive of the fibrous origin of the tumour.
  - Tumours tend to be related to the deep fascia.
  - Extension into the surrounding soft tissues and cortical destruction of the adjacent bone are frequent findings.
- Due to its aggressive nature, prognosis for a patient with adult-type fibrosarcoma is guarded. Many factors come into play including extent of invasion at time of diagnosis, resection margins and response to chemotherapy etc.
- Our case (Figure 4.15) was unusual as the tumour was superficially located, though still in relation to fascia, and did not invade adjacent structures. Imaging features mimicked nodular fasciitis. On histology, there were no features of dermatofibrosarcoma protuberans or of myxofibrosarcoma – differentials for superficially located fibrous tumours.

● *Myxofibrosarcoma*

- Tends to afflict patients in their fifth or sixth decade of life.
- Has a predilection for the dermal and subcutaneous tissues of lower limbs (as opposed to deeper soft tissues for other aggressive soft tissue sarcomas).
- MRI: Lesions invariably demonstrate abnormal signal and infiltration along the fascial plane with tail-like tumour margins (**refer to orange arrows in** Figure 4.16) extending into

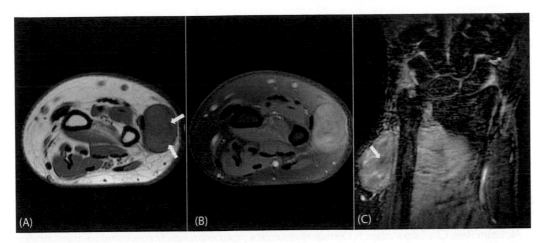

Figure 4.15: Low-grade fibrosarcoma in a 50-year-old male patient presenting with rapidly enlarging wrist lump. A fairly well-marginated T1 hypointense (A), moderately enhancing (B) and T2 heterogeneous, predominantly hypointense with T2 hyperintensities (C) soft tissue tumour is seen in the subcutaneous tissues of distal forearm. Note the relation of tumour to the fascia and band-like areas of low signal intensity on T1W and T2W images suggestive of fibrous origin of tumour (arrows).

surrounding tissues for a substantial distance. The myxoid component of the tumour shows T1 hypointensity and T2 bright signal intensity and shows relatively less enhancement when compared to the non-myxoid component.

- Myxofibrosarcomas, like other high-grade sarcomas, have a propensity to metastasise to the lungs.
- A study showed a five-year survival rate of 63% which is better compared to other soft tissue sarcomas.

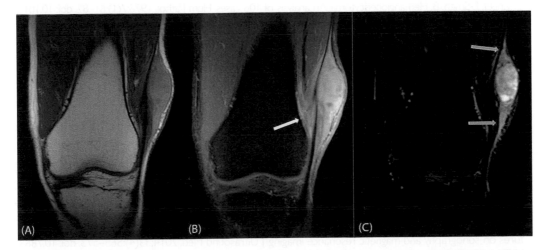

Figure 4.16: Myxofibrosarcoma of thigh in a 49-year-old female. Coronal T1W pre- and post-contrast (A and B, respectively) and coronal fluid-sensitive STIR (C) sequences show a large infiltrative superficially spreading mass showing avid post-contrast enhancement. Note the fascial tail sign (orange arrows) as well as deep infiltration in the vastus lateralis muscle (yellow arrow).

Take-home points

- WHO classification categorises fibrous, myofibroblastic and fibrohistiocytic tumours as benign, intermediate (locally aggressive), intermediate (rarely metastasising) and malignant.
- MRI remains the mainstay of imaging modality, although ultrasound, computed radiography and CT can be helpful in some cases.
- Knowledge about these tumours and their imaging-specific appearances especially on MRI can shorten the list of differential diagnoses.
- Determining the local extent of disease, its relationship to surrounding structures and post-treatment surveillance are key roles of the radiologist.

SUGGESTED READING

- Alcántara Reifs, CM, Salido-Vallejo, R. Dermatofibrosarcoma protuberans with fibrosarcomatous transformation. An Bras Dermatol. 2016;91(5):700–701. doi: 10.1590/ABD1806-4841.20164886.
- Amendola, MA, Glazer, GM, Agha, FP, Francis, IR, Weatherbee, L, Martel, W. Myositis ossificans circumscripta: Computed tomographic diagnosis. Radiology. 1983;149(3 I):775–779. doi: 10.1148/RADIOLOGY.149.3.6647854.
- Augsburger, D, Nelson, PJ, Kalinski, T, et al. Current diagnostics and treatment of fibrosarcoma: Perspectives for future therapeutic targets and strategies. Oncotarget. 2017;8(61):104638–104653. doi: 10.18632/ONCOTARGET.20136.
- Bansal, A, Goyal, S, Goyal, A, Jana, M. WHO classification of soft tissue tumours 2020: An update and simplified approach for radiologists. Eur J Radiol. 2021;143(82):109937. doi: 10.1016/j.ejrad.2021.109937.
- Clarke, L, Zhang, P, Crawford, G, Elenitsas, R. Myxofibrosarcoma in the skin. J Cutan Pathol. 2008;35(10): 935–940. doi: 10.1111/J.1600-0560.2007.00922.X.
- Coffin, C, Dehner, L. Fibroblastic-myofibroblastic tumors in children and adolescents: A clinicopathologic study of 108 examples in 103 patients. Pediatr Pathol. 1991;11(4):569–588. doi: 10.3109/15513819109064791.
- Coyle, J, White, LM, Dickson, B, Ferguson, P, Wunder, J, Naraghi, A. MRI characteristics of nodular fasciitis of the musculoskeletal system. Skelet Radiol. 2013;42(7):975–982. doi: 10.1007/S00256-013-1620-9.
- Darwish, FM, Haddad, W. Giant cell tumour of tendon sheath: Experience with 52 cases. Singapore Med J. 2008;49(11):879.
- Dewan, V, Darbyshire, A, Sumathi, V, Jeys, L, Grimer, R. Prognostic and survival factors in myxofibrosarcomas. Sarcoma. 2012;2012. doi: 10.1155/2012/830879.
- Enzinger, F, Smith, B. Hemangiopericytoma. An analysis of 106 cases. Hum Pathol. 1976;7(1):61–82. doi: 10.1016/S0046-8177(76)80006-8.
- Erickson-Johnson, MR, Chou, MM, Evers, BR, et al. Nodular fasciitis: A novel model of transient neoplasia induced by MYH9-USP6 gene fusion. Lab Invest. 2011;91(10):1427–1433. doi: 10.1038/LABINVEST.2011.118.
- Ferrari, A, Alaggio, R, Meazza, C, et al. Fibroblastic tumors of intermediate malignancy in childhood. Expert Rev Anticancer Ther. 2014;13(2):225–236. doi: 10.1586/ERA.12.180.
- Fletcher CD, Unni KK, Mertens F, editors. Pathology and genetics of tumours of soft tissue and bone. Lyon, France: Iarc; 2002.
- Fox, M, Kransdorf, M, Bancroft, L, Peterson, J, Flemming, D. MR imaging of fibroma of the tendon sheath. AJR Am J Roentgenol. 2003;180(5):1449–1453. doi: 10.2214/AJR.180.5.1801449.
- Goldblum, J, Weiss, S, Folpe, AL. Enzinger and Weiss's soft tissue tumors. 7th ed. Elsevier; 2019.
- Goni, V, Gopinathan, N, Radotra, B, Viswanathan, V, Logithasan, R. S B. Giant cell tumour of peroneus brevis tendon sheath: A case report and review of literature. BMJ Case Rep. 2012;2012. doi: 10.1136/BCR.01.2012.5703.
- Harrill, J, Johnston, R. Plexiform fibrohistiocytic tumor of the foot: A case report. J Foot Ankle Surg. 2014;53(5):635–637. doi: 10.1053/J.JFAS.2014.02.006.
- Khuu, A, Yablon, C, Jacobson, J, Inyang, A, Lucas, D, Biermann, J. Nodular fasciitis: Characteristic imaging features on sonography and magnetic resonance imaging. J Ultrasound Med. 2014;33(4):565–573. doi: 10.7863/ULTRA.33.4.565.
- Kim, SJ, Kim, WS, Cheon, J-E, et al. Inflammatory myofibroblastic tumors of the abdomen as mimickers of malignancy: Imaging features in nine children. Am J Roentgenol. 2012;193(5):1419–1424. doi: 10.2214/AJR.09.2433.
- Kransdorf, MJ, Murphey, MD. Imaging of soft tissue tumours. 3rd ed. Lippincott Williams and Wilkins; 2013.
- Kransdorff, MJ, Meis-Kindblom, JM. Dermatofibrosarcoma protuberans: Radiologic appearance. AJR Am J Roentgenol. Published online 1994. Accessed December 22, 2021. www.ajronline.org

- Massengill, A, Sundaram, M, Kathol, M, El-Khoury, G, Buckwalter, J, Wade, T. Elastofibroma dorsi: A radiological diagnosis. Skeletal Radiol. 1993;22(2):121–123. doi: 10.1007/BF00197991.
- Meister, P, Bückmann, F, Konrad, E. Nodular fasciitis (analysis of 100 cases and review of the literature). Pathol Res Pract. 1978;162(2):133–165. doi: 10.1016/S0344-0338(78)80001-6.
- Miettinen, M, Fetsch, J. Collagenous fibroma (desmoplastic fibroblastoma): A clinicopathologic analysis of 63 cases of a distinctive soft tissue lesion with stellate-shaped fibroblasts. Hum Pathol. 1998;29(7):676–682. doi: 10.1016/S0046-8177(98)90275-1.
- Järvi, OH, Länsimies, PH, L. Subclinical elastofibromas in the scapular region in an autopsy series. Acta Pathol Microbiol Scand A. 1975;83(1):87–108. doi: 10.1111/J.1699-0463.1975.TB01361.X.
- Oweis, Y, Lucas, D, Brandon, C, Girish, G, Jacobson, J, Fessell, D. Extra-abdominal desmoid tumor with osseous involvement. Skeletal Radiol. 2012;41(4):483–487. doi: 10.1007/S00256-011-1336-7.
- Patel, RM, Singh, R, Udager, AM, Billings, SD. Benign fibrous, fibrohistiocytic, and myofibroblastic lesions. In: Billings SD, Patel RM, Buehler D, eds. Soft tissue tumors of the skin. New York: Springer; 2019, pp. 91–174. doi:10.1007/978-1-4939-8812-9_4.
- Patnana, M, Sevrukov, AB, Elsayes, KM, Viswanathan, C, Lubner, M, Menias, CO. Inflammatory pseudotumor: The great mimicker. Am J Roentgenol. 2012;198(3). doi:10.2214/AJR.11.7288.
- Peh, W, TShek, T, Ip, W. Growing wrist mass. Ann Rheum Dis. 2001;60(6):550–553. doi: 10.1136/ARD.60.6.550.
- Roberts, CC, Liu, PT, Chew, FS. Imaging evaluation of tendon sheath disease: Self-assessment module. Am J Roentgenol. 2012;188(3 SUPPL. 1). doi: 10.2214/AJR.06.1484.
- Sargar, KM, Sheybani, EF, Shenoy, A, Aranake-Chrisinger, J, Khanna, G. Pediatric fibroblastic and myofibroblastic tumors: A pictorial review. Radiographics. 2016;36(4):1195–1214. doi: 10.1148/RG.2016150191.
- Sbaraglia, M, Bellan, E, Dei Tos, AP. The 2020 WHO classification of soft tissue tumours: News and perspectives. Pathologica. 2021;113(2):70–84. doi: 10.32074/1591-951X-213.
- Shinagare, AB, Ramaiya, NH, Jagannathan, JP, et al. A to Z of desmoid tumors. Am J Clin Pathol. 2012;197(6). doi: 10.2214/AJR.11.6657.
- Subramanian, S, Sharma, R. Can MR imaging be used to reliably differentiate proliferative myositis from myositis ossificans? Radiology. 2008;246(3):987. doi: 10.1148/RADIOL.2463071346.
- Suresh, SS, Zaki, H. Giant cell tumor of tendon sheath: Case series and review of literature. J Hand Microsurg. 2010;2(2):67. doi: 10.1007/S12593-010-0020-9.
- Tyler, P, Saifuddin, A. The imaging of myositis ossificans. Semin Musculoskelet Radiol. 2010;14(2):201–216. doi: 10.1055/s-0030-1253161.
- Walker, KR, Bui-Mansfield, LT, Gering, SA, Ranlett, RD. Collagenous fibroma (desmoplastic fibroblastoma) of the shoulder. Am J Roentgenol. 2012;183(6):1766. doi: 10.2214/AJR.183.6.01831766.
- Walker, EA, Petscavage, JM, Brian, PL, Logie, CI, Montini, KM, Murphey, MD. Imaging features of superficial and deep fibromatoses in the adult population. Sarcoma. 2012;2012:17. doi: 10.1155/2012/215810.
- WHO Classification of Tumours Editorial Board W. Soft tissue and bone tumours. In: WHO classification of tumours, Vol 3. 5th ed. International Agency for Research on Cancer; 2020.
- Wignall, O, Moskovic, E, Thway, K, Thomas, J. Solitary fibrous tumors of the soft tissues: Review of the imaging and clinical features with histopathologic correlation. AJR Am J Roentgenol. 2010;195(1):W55–62. doi: 10.2214/AJR.09.3379.
- Yamamoto, A, Abe, S, Imamura, T, et al. Three cases of collagenous fibroma with rim enhancement on postcontrast T1-weighted images with fat suppression. Skeletal Radiol. 2013;42(1):141–146. doi: 10.1007/S00256-012-1484-4.
- Yu, J. Pathologic and post-operative conditions of the plantar fascia: Review of MR imaging appearances. Skeletal Radiol. 2000;29(9):491–501. doi: 10.1007/S002560000230.

5 Peripheral nerve tumours

Abhinav Bansal, Ankur Goyal

INTRODUCTION

Peripheral nerve sheath tumours represent a heterogenous group of soft tissue neoplasms which arise from the neuroectoderm. They are rare in the general population, with benign tumours being more common than the malignant counterparts. Neurofibroma and schwannoma are the most common benign tumours which may occur sporadically or in association with neurofibromatosis. Malignant peripheral nerve sheath tumours (MPNST) generally occur in association with neurofibromatosis type 1 (NF1) (40–60% cases). They are the sixth most common soft tissue sarcomas with an incidence of 1:100,000 in the general population. Patients with NF1 have an increased lifetime risk of developing MPNST with an incidence of 1:3500.

Peripheral nerve sheath tumours were included in the World Health Organisation (WHO) classification for the first time in 2013. Apart from neurofibroma and schwannoma, other benign entities in this group include perineuroma, granular cell tumour, nerve sheath myxoma and hybrid nerve sheath tumours (Table 5.1). Malignant melanotic nerve sheath tumour, previously known as melanotic schwannoma has been added to the category of malignant tumours in the recent 2020 revision of WHO classification after recognition of its aggressive behaviour. Other malignant entities include MPNSTs and malignant perineuroma (Table 5.1).

Table 5.1: WHO Classification of Peripheral Nerve Sheath Tumours

Benign
Schwannoma
Neurofibroma
Plexiform neurofibroma
Perineurioma
Granular cell tumour
Nerve sheath myxoma
Solitary circumscribed neuroma
Meningioma
Malignant
Malignant peripheral nerve sheath tumour
Melanotic malignant nerve sheath tumour
Malignant granular cell tumour
Malignant perineurioma

DOI: 10.1201/9781003218722-5

Radiologists play a vital role in diagnosis by suggesting the neural origin of these neoplasms. Also, true tumours can be differentiated from pseudotumours such as traumatic neuroma, Morton's neuroma and intramural ganglia. Imaging further helps in identification of suspicious features to detect malignant lesions and also provides appropriate route for image-guided biopsy.

IMAGING MODALITIES

● *Ultrasound*

Ultrasound is commonly used initial modality of choice for superficially located palpable lesions. Due to its high spatial and contrast resolution, it can demonstrate the major peripheral nerves in relation to the tumour.

- It also differentiates solid from cystic lesions and is helpful in assessing presence of internal vascularity.
- It can also be used for image-guided biopsy of the lesions. However, it provides limited evaluation of deep-seated lesions and is operator-dependent.
- A normal nerve has hypoechoic nerve fascicles against a background of echogenic connective tissue giving it a honeycomb appearance in transverse section (Figure 5.1).
- Tumours appear as hypoechoic masses in relation to a nerve with variable internal vascularity.

● *Computed tomography scan*

Computed tomography (CT) has limited role in evaluation of peripheral nerve tumours.

- It is usually employed for assessing lesions located in head and neck region, mediastinum and retroperitoneum.
- Positron emission tomography (PET) combined with CT can provide functional information for differentiating benign from malignant tumours (Figure 5.2). Maximum standard uptake value (SUV_{max}) of more than 3 and high SUV on delayed scans are associated with malignant lesions.

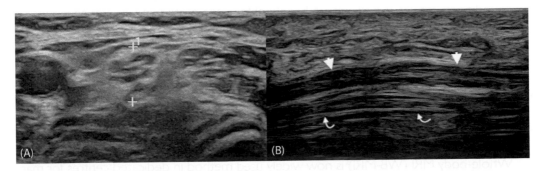

Figure 5.1: Normal ultrasound architecture of the peripheral nerve. (A) Short-axis greyscale ultrasound image shows hypoechoic nerve fascicles separated by hyperechoic interstitial fat giving "honeycomb" appearance. (B) Long-axis greyscale image shows coarse fibrillar pattern of a nerve (arrow heads – median nerve) compared to finer fibrillar pattern of an underlying flexor tendon (curved arrows).

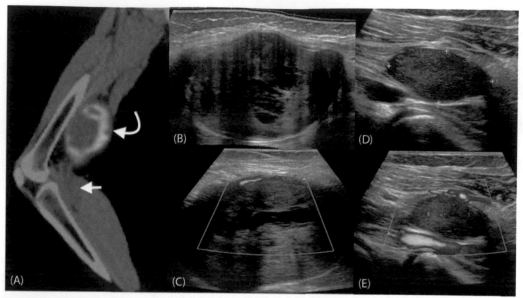

Figure 5.2: Use of positron emission tomography-computed tomography (PET-CT). (A) Sagittal reconstruction of a fused PET-CT image shows a large soft tissue mass lesion in the sciatic nerve showing intense peripheral uptake (SUV max more than 3, curved arrow) which was diagnosed MPNST on the ultrasound-guided biopsy and smaller lesion within the tibial nerve consistent with benign neurofibroma (low tracer uptake, straight arrow). (B) Greyscale and (C) colour Doppler images show typical ultrasound features of the MPNST a large (more than 5 cm) with necrotic components and increased vascularity. Compares the ultrasound features with (D) greyscale and (E) colour Doppler images of the benign neurofibroma which show small, solid lesion with increased vascularity. (Image Courtesy of Dr Siddharth Thaker.)

● *Magnetic resonance imaging*

Magnetic resonance imaging (MRI) is the imaging gold standard for evaluation of peripheral nerve tumours.

- It better characterizes the intratumoural morphology, vascularity and relation to surrounding structures. It is also more beneficial for deep-seated and infiltrating lesions.
- MRI can also provide useful clues for differentiating benign from malignant lesions. Larger size (>5 cm) with presence of central necrosis and peripheral post-contrast enhancement are suspicious features seen more commonly in malignant tumours (Figure 5.3).
- Denervation changes can be better appreciated on MRI.
- T2-weighted sequence should be performed in all three planes with fat-saturated sequence in at least one plane.
- Diffusion-weighted imaging (DWI) (Figure 5.4) and post-contrast images are capable of providing additional useful information.
- Whole-body MRI (WB-MRI) is now widely used method in dedicated centres for management of genetically or clinically proven NF. WB-MRI is useful in establishing disease burden (Figure 5.5), assessing changes in size and signal characteristics of "at-risk" lesions for sarcomatous differentiation and detecting additional neural crest tumours. WB-MRI and whole-spine MRI can depict scoliosis, dural ectasia, plexiform neurofibromata, secondary soft tissue and bony changes in the vertebral column and skull (Figure 5.6).

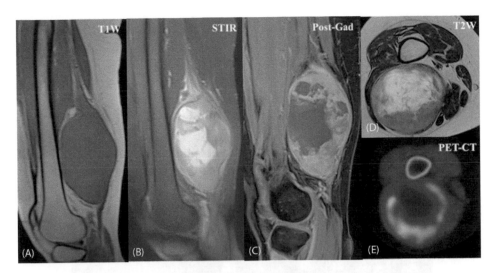

Figure 5.3: Utility of MRI in the MPNST. Various MRI sequences taken to evaluate an MPNST described in Figure 5.2. (A) T1-weighted sagittal image shows the sciatic nerve entering and exiting a large tumour which shows extensive heterogeneity on sagittal STIR (B), extensive internal necrosis on post-gadolinium (C) and axial T2-weighted (D) images and intense peripheral radiotracer uptake (E) along with rapid growth are characteristic findings of a sarcomatous transformation (MPNST). (Image Courtesy of Dr Siddharth Thaker.)

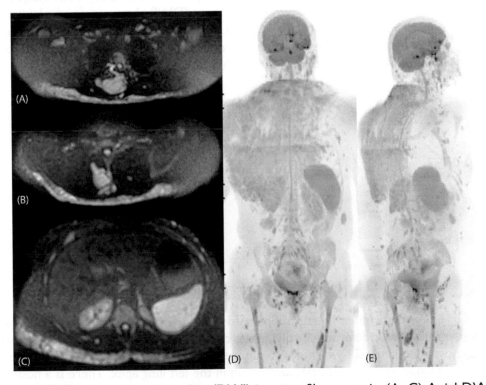

Figure 5.4: Diffusion-weighted imaging (DWI) in neurofibromatosis. (A–C) Axial DWI and (D and E) 3D-reconstructed DWI show a large plaque-like neurofibroma, plexiform posterior paravertebral neurofibroma and additional innumerable superficial and deep neurofibromata. (Image Courtesy of Dr Siddharth Thaker.)

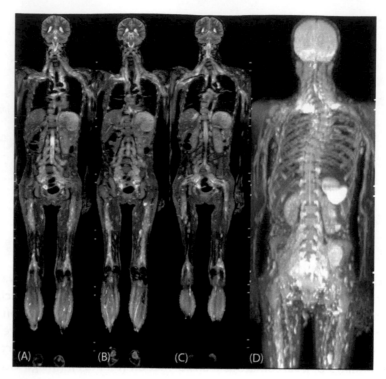

Figure 5.5: Whole-body MRI in neurofibromatosis. (A–C) Whole-body STIR images and (D) 3D-reconstructed diffusion-weighted images (DWI) show extensive plexiform neurofibroma involving both brachial and lumbosacral plexuses and cord-like thickening of upper and lower limb peripheral nerves bilaterally. Also appreciate cervicothoracic kyphosis on DWI. (Image Courtesy of Dr Siddharth Thaker.)

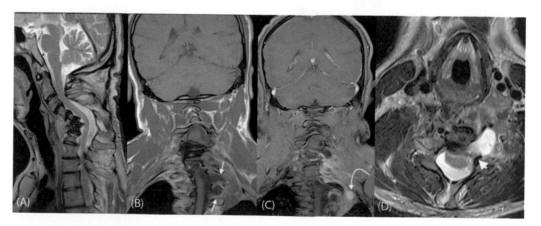

Figure 5.6: Spinal deformities in neurofibromatosis type 1. (A) T2-weighted sagittal image shows severe kyphotic deformity involving the cervical spine, (B) T1-weighted coronal and (C) post-gadolinium T1-weighted fat-suppressed images show dural ectasia (arrows) and a large plaque-like neurofibromatous tissue in the left lung apex. There is a nodular enhancement (curved) along the left C8 nerve root which presents an "at-risk" lesion that can be followed up. (D) T2-weighted axial image showing bony (widened neural exit foramen – arrow head) and soft tissue deformities. (Image Courtesy of Dr Siddharth Thaker.)

BENIGN NEUROGENIC TUMOURS

● *Neurofibromas*

These tumours are composed of differentiated Schwann cells, perineurial cells, fibroblasts and interspersed axons embedded in a myxoid and collagenous extracellular matrix. Neurofibromas commonly occur in the younger population (20–30 years) and multiple tumours can occur in paraspinal location in NF1.

Three morphological types are described: localised, diffuse and plexiform.

- *Localized:* Majority of the lesions (90%) are of the localised variety (Figure 5.7). These usually occur in skin and subcutaneous tissue with only occasional involvement of deep nerves. Superficial lesions present as painless nodules whereas deeper ones can have associated neurological symptoms.
- *Diffuse:* These are uncommon lesions which predominantly occur in children and young adults. They usually involve the skin and subcutaneous tissue of head and neck and cause plaque-like thickening of the involved tissues (Figure 5.8). The extent can be so extensive along the connective tissues that it may lead to gigantism of an extremity.

Majority of localised and diffuse neurofibromas are not associated with NF1.

- *Plexiform neurofibromas:* These are pathognomic of NF1. These occur in early childhood. There is diffuse long segment enlargement of a nerve and its branches, giving a gross appearance of "bag of worms". These lesions typically have a multilobulated tubular morphology (Figure 5.9) and may invade surrounding soft tissues.

Neurofibromas grow in a fusiform manner with the involved nerve entering and exiting from the lesion (Figure 5.10). They do not have a surrounding capsule; therefore, surgical excision requires sacrificing the parent nerve in most of the cases. Since neoplastic component is Schwann cell, thus on staining for S100 and SOX10, immunoreactivity is seen, though not as extensive as in schwannomas. CD 34 positivity is seen in the stromal component and is usually more pronounced than in schwannomas.

Ultrasound is non-specific but usually shows hypoechoic nodular lesions with surrounding hyperechogenicity. Posterior acoustic enhancement has also been reported. These

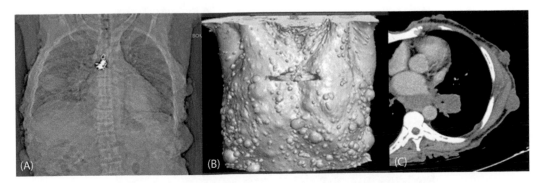

Figure 5.7: Multiple skin and subcutaneous, along with mediastinal and hilar localised, neurofibromas. (A) Topogram and (B) volume-rendered image (VRT) showing multiple skin and subcutaneous lesions (white arrows). (C) Axial CT image showing mediastinal and left hilar neurofibromas (white arrows) along with subcutaneous lesions.

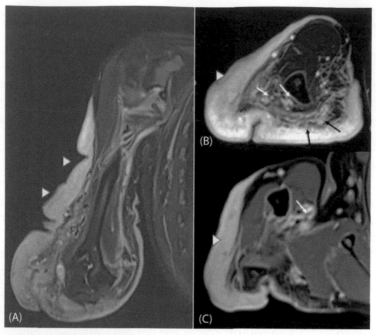

Figure 5.8: Superficial and deep diffuse plaque-like neurofibromas in (A) coronal and (B) axial T2-weighted fat-suppressed images show diffuse T2 hyperintense involvement of the cutaneous subcutaneous tissues (arrow heads) in the arm with thickening of the nerve fascicles (white arrows in B) along with atrophy of the muscles (black arrows in b). (C) Post-contrast T1-weighted fat-suppressed image showing enhancement of the subcutaneous masses (arrow head) and the nerve fascicles (white arrow).

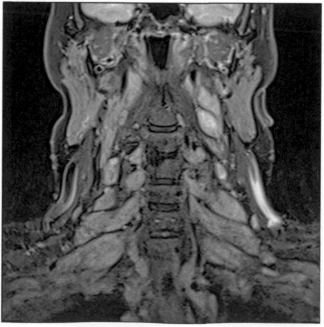

Figure 5.9: Plexiform neurofibroma. Extensive neurofibroma involving entire brachial plexus on both sides and cervical nerves giving "bag-of-worms" appearance. (Image Courtesy of Dr Siddharth Thaker.)

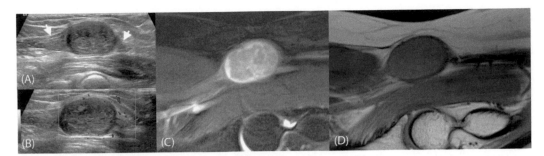

Figure 5.10: Neurofibroma. (A) Greyscale and (B) colour Doppler images showing fusiform enlargement of the median nerve where the nerve enters and exits (arrows) into the well-encapsuled solid mass lesion – tail sign. Corresponding (C) STIR and (D) T1-weighted images confirm features of peripheral nerve sheath tumour consistent with neurofibroma. (Image Courtesy of Dr Siddharth Thaker.)

lesions may have a pseudocystic appearance because of marked hypoechogenicity and posterior acoustic enhancement. However, there are no compressible cystic spaces. Internal colour vascularity is variable. Sonographic target sign has also been described with echogenic central part and hypoechoic peripheral area. Echogenic ring like appearance may also be seen.

They are seen as oblong lesions on CT, which are hypodense relative to surrounding muscle and show little post-contrast enhancement.

On MRI, following characteristic features are described:

- *Target sign:* On T2W images, central T2 hypointensity is seen corresponding to collagen and fibrillary core with peripheral T2 hyperintensity due to myxoid tissue, giving a target appearance (Figure 5.11). Similarly, on post-contrast imaging central enhancement is seen with peripheral hypointensity (also termed as the reverse target sign).
- *Fascicular sign:* Multiple curvilinear T2 hypointense foci are seen in background of T2 hyperintense areas, corresponding to the presence of nerve fascicles (Figure 5.10).
- *Split fat sign:* This refers to presence of fat at upper and lower pole of the lesion on a T1-weighted image (Figure 5.12), representing intermuscular location of the tumour. It is a feature of benignity and can be seen in any soft tissue tumour arising in intermuscular location like myxoma.
- *Muscular atrophy:* Atrophy of muscles with fatty replacement may be seen in the distribution of affected nerve (Figure 5.8).
- T2 hyperintense rim and tumoural cysts are more commonly seen in schwannomas.

● *Schwannoma*

Schwannomas (also called neurilemoma) are encapsulated lesions consisting of differentiated neoplastic Schwann cells that occur in age group of 30–50 years. They are usually slow-growing painless masses that cause symptoms only due to compression of neighbouring structures. Spinal and sympathetic nerves of head and neck and major nerve trunks are commonly affected sites (Figure 5.12). Paraspinal dumbbell-shaped lesions (intraspinal and extraspinal component with constriction at the level of neural foramen) can also occur (Figure 5.13), especially in NF2. Bilateral vestibular schwannomas are pathognomic for

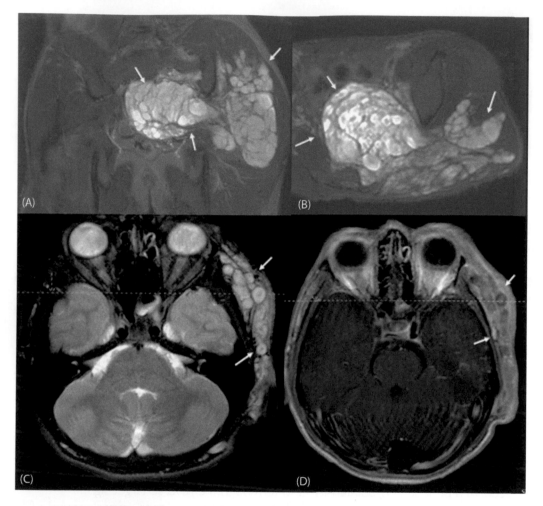

Figure 5.11: Plexiform neurofibroma. (A) Coronal and (B) axial T2-weighted images show infiltrative lesion with T2 hyperintense tubular structures within and having peripheral T2 hyperintensity and central less T2 hyperintense region (target sign) in the pelvis and left gluteal region along the course of sciatic nerve (white arrows). (C) Axial T2 fat-suppressed image of a different patient showing an infiltrative subcutaneous T2 hyperintense lesion with target sign within in left temporal region (white arrows). (D) Axial post-contrast T1 fat-suppressed image showing central enhancement within the tubular structures (white arrows) with peripheral non-enhancing area (reverse target sign).

NF2. Multiple schwannomas can also occur in Schwannomatosis but occur in adulthood in contrast to NF2 where they tend to occur early (Figure 5.14).

Schwannomas arise within the nerve sheath; therefore, they are eccentrically located in relation to nerve (Figure 5.15). They are contained within a true capsule which makes separation from the parent nerve possible during surgery. The tumours show diffuse nuclear and cytoplasmic staining for S100 and SOX10 immunoreactivity. Giant schwannomas (>10 cm) are rare but may occur in the lumbosacral region. The histological subtypes include ancient, cellular, plexiform, epithelioid and reticular/microcystic types. Ancient schwannomas

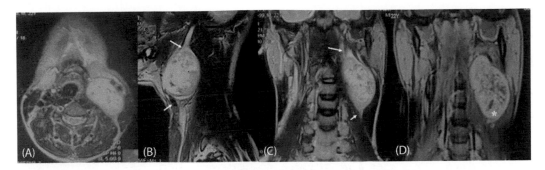

Figure 5.12: Vagal schwannoma. (A) Axial, (B) sagittal and (C) coronal T2-weighted images show heterogenous T2 hyperintense mass within the left carotid space with displacement of carotid artery and jugular vein anteriorly and "split fat sign" (white arrows) at upper and lower poles. The lesion shows a T2 hyperintense rim. (D) Coronal post-contrast T1 fat-saturated image showing heterogenous enhancement within the tumour (asterix).

are long-standing lesions which have internal calcification, hyalinisation and cystic areas representing degenerative changes.

The sonographic appearance of schwannoma is similar to neurofibroma. These lesions are longitudinally ovoid in shape, hypoechoic, show internal heterogencity and may be seen in relation to a major nerve (Figure 5.15).

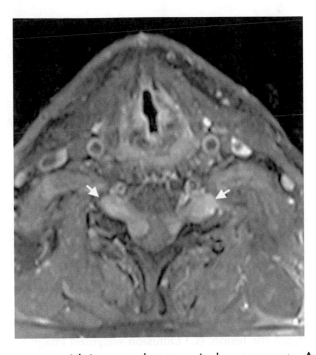

Figure 5.13: Schwannomas with intra- and extra-spinal components. Adult-onset schwannomatosis patient shows dumbbell-shaped enhancing schwannomas (arrows) with intra- and extra-spinal components on a contrast-enhanced T1-weighted fat-suppressed image. Intradural components show marked spinal compression. (Image Courtesy of Dr Siddharth Thaker.)

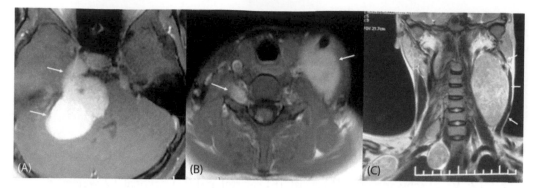

Figure 5.14: Neurofibromatosis 2. Axial post-contrast MRI (A) depict bilateral trigeminal nerve schwannomas with extension to right Meckel's cave (white arrows). Post-contrast image at a lower section (B) shows schwannomas in right neural foramen and left carotid sheath location (white arrows). (C) Coronal T2-weighted image demonstrates multiple longitudinally ovoid lesions in paraspinal, carotid sheath and along the right brachial plexus (white arrows).

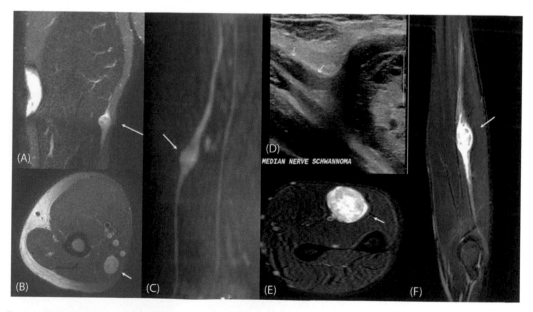

Figure 5.15: Ulnar and median nerve schwannomas. (A) Coronal and (B) axial T2-weighted images show T2 hyperintense tumour (white arrows) located in the posterior medial aspect of arm along the course of ulnar nerve with nerve seen entering and exiting from the lesion. (C) Diffusion-weighted image with background suppression (DWIBS) shows the tumour (white arrows) in continuity with the ulnar nerve. Different patient: (D) Ultrasound image shows a mixed echoic mass present eccentrically along the median nerve (white arrows). (E) Axial and (F) coronal T2 fat-suppressed images show T2 hyperintense tumour (white arrow) located eccentrically along the median nerve in forearm.

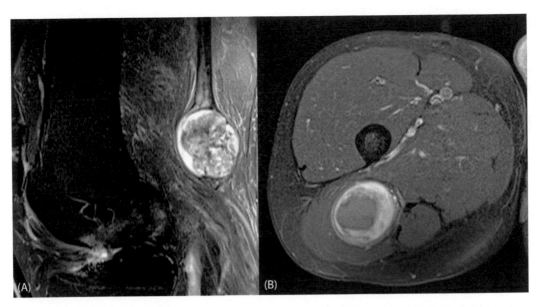

Figure 5.16: MRI appearances of neurofibroma versus schwannoma. (A) Sagittal STIR image shows a solid heterogenous lesion in the course of the sciatic nerve. The lesion is located centrally. (B) Gadolinium-enhanced T1-weighted fat-suppressed axial image shows a large necrotic eccentrically located lesion in the course of the sciatic nerve – biopsy proven schwannoma. (Image Courtesy of Dr. Harun Gupta.)

On CT, well-defined hypodense lesion is seen which shows post-contrast enhancement with internal cystic areas. Scalloping in surrounding bones may be seen due to mass effect.

On MRI, schwannomas are hypointense on T1W and hyperintense on T2W images with internal cystic areas. Larger lesions have more heterogenous appearance due to degeneration and haemorrhage.

- T2 hyperintense rim sign can be seen around the lesion. It is more common in schwannomas as compared to neurofibroma (Figure 5.16).
- Target sign is also seen in schwannomas due to the presence of more cellular Antoni A cells in the centre with a surrounding rim of less cellular Antoni B cells.

Malignant degeneration is rare in schwannomas and local recurrence does not occur if completely excised. The distinction between schwannoma and neurofibroma is difficult because of overlapping imaging features; nevertheless, some helpful points are listed in Table 5.2.

Table 5.2: Differentiating Features Between Schwannoma and Neurofibroma

Schwannoma	Neurofibroma
Eccentric in relation to nerve	Centred within the nerve with involvement of nerve fascicles
True capsule present	True capsule absent
Heterogenous with cystic changes	Relatively homogenous
T2 hyperintense rim more common	Less common
Fascicular sign not seen	Fascicular sign present
Can be separated from parent nerve during surgery	Separation from parent nerve usually not possible during surgery
Associated with neurofibromatosis type 2	Associated with neurofibromatosis type 1

● *Other benign nerve sheath tumours*

Perineuriomas occur in the extremities and trunk. Granular cell tumours commonly occur in the tongue and breasts. Dermal nerve sheath myxomas occur in the distal extremities, particularly involving the fingers/toes.

MALIGNANT NEUROGENIC TUMOURS

● *Malignant peripheral nerve sheath tumours*

They represent 5–10% of soft tissue sarcomas. Majority of the tumours (50%) occur in association with NF1. They generally involve the major nerve trunks with soft tissue mass, pain and neurological deficits being the presenting symptoms. Secondary malignant degeneration can occur due to prior radiation therapy with a latency period of more than 10 years. They are commonly seen as large fusiform masses on imaging with internal necrosis and haemorrhage (Figure 5.17).

Features favouring malignancy include:
- Large size more than 5 cm
- Ill-defined infiltrative margins with surrounding oedema
- Heterogeneity with central necrosis, cystic areas and haemorrhage
- Peripheral nodular enhancement
- Perilesional oedema-like zone
- Intraosseous lytic lesions with cortical destruction and associated soft tissue in setting of NF1.
- Diffusion restriction on diffusion-weighted MRI
- On PET, higher standard uptake values (SUV) are seen in MPNST as compared to schwannomas and neurofibromas.

● *Malignant melanotic nerve sheath tumours*

These were previously known as melanotic schwannoma. They have been reclassified in the malignant subgroup in the recent WHO classification due to recognition of aggressive nature. They affect the adult population and tend to involve the midline autonomic and spinal nerves. They are associated with Carney complex with a younger age of onset in this subgroup.

● *Neurofibromatosis*

NF1, also known as Von Recklinghausen disease, is an autosomal disorder that occurs due to mutation of NF1 gene on chromosome 17q11.2. This disease is characterized by multiple neurofibromas, optic pathway gliomas, sphenoid wing dysplasia, café-au-lait spots, axillary/inguinal freckling and pigmented iris nodules. Localised dermal neurofibromas occur on the trunk in 95% of cases, ranging in size from 1 mm up to 2 cm. Diffuse subcutaneous neurofibromas are less common.

Plexiform neurofibromas are pathognomic for NF1 developing in 30 to 50% individuals. They are bulky, infiltrating, rope-like tumours associated with major nerve trunks and branches. Of these, 10 to 15% can have malignant transformation, more commonly in deep-seated lesions.

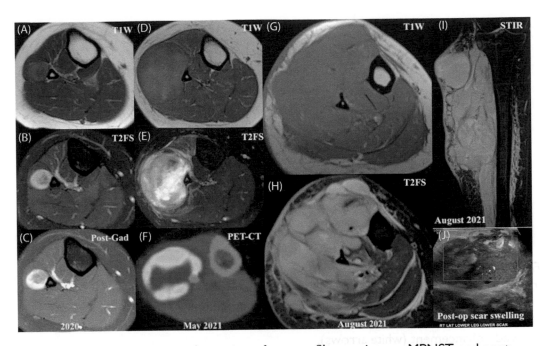

Figure 5.17: Sarcomatous transformation of a neurofibroma into an MPNST and post-operative recurrence. The patient has initially presented in late 2020 with mild symptoms. (A) T1-weighted, (B) T2-weighted fat-suppressed and (C) gadolinium-enhanced images show a small PNST arising from the common peroneal nerve. The patient was placed under close clinical and imaging surveillance. Six-months follow-up MRI shows marked increase in the tumour volume, permeative marrow involvement of the fibular shaft and denervation oedema involving the anterior and lateral compartment muscles on (D) T1-weighted and (E) T2-weighted fat-suppressed images. Pre-operative imaging work-up with PET-CT (F) shows typical sarcomatous tracer uptake. There was a delay in surgical treatment and up-to-date immediate pre-operative MRI shows explosive growth of the MPNST with multicompartment involvement on (G) T1-weighted, (H) T2-weighted fat-suppressed axial and (I) STIR coronal image and secondary muscle changes. The patient had above knee amputation and within weeks presented with enlarging swelling at the scar site. (J) Colour Doppler ultrasound image demonstrates solid soft tissue mass at the scar with disorganised internal vascularity consistent with scar site recurrence. (Image Courtesy of Dr. Harun Gupta.)

DIFFERENTIAL DIAGNOSES

- *Venous malformations:* Venous malformations are the most common differential of nerve sheath tumours. The common features include skin pigmentation, hypoechoic appearance on ultrasound, T2 hyperintensity and tubular morphology (Figure 5.18). Moreover, the target sign may be mistaken for phleboliths and both show heterogeneous enhancement on delayed post-contrast images. Differentiating features include solid nature (versus cystic appearing compressible lesion in venous malformations) and gradually progressive filling of the spaces on dynamic post-contrast images in venous malformations.
- *Lymphatic malformations:* Like nerve sheath tumours, these appear hypodense on CT. On ultrasound, the hypoechogenicity of nerve sheath tumours may sometimes be mistaken for anechoic nature of lymphatic malformations, especially because the former may also be associated with posterior acoustic enhancement. Microcystic lymphatic

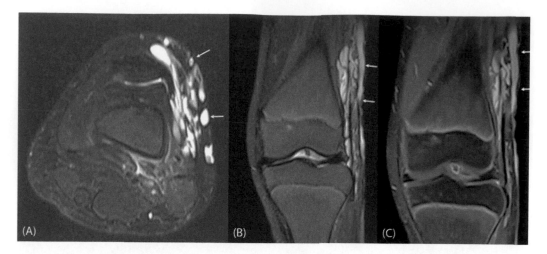

Figure 5.18: Venous malformation. (A) Axial and (B) coronal T2-weighted fat-suppressed images showing multiple T2 hyperintense cystic and tubular structures within the subcutaneous plane (white arrows) on medial aspect of lower thigh and knee joint. (C) Coronal post-contrast T1-weighted fat-suppressed image showing homogenous delayed enhancement (white arrows).

malformation may sometimes require sampling to differentiate from soft tissue neo-plasms like nerve sheath tumours.

- *Myxoma:* These also appear brightly hyperintense on T2W images, show heterogeneous enhancement and may show polar fat sign.
- Other soft tissue tumours like angiofibroma, tenosynovial giant cell tumour and rhabdomyoma.

CONCLUSIONS

Of the soft tissue tumours, nerve sheath tumours are the only category in which origin is neuroectoderm rather than the mesoderm. These are relatively easy to diagnose, though difficulty arises in detecting malignant change. Relationship to a nerve trunk and various signs on MRI aid in making the correct diagnosis.

Take-home points

- Nerve sheath tumours have a characteristic longitudinally oval or dumbbell shape.
- Target sign, fascicular sign and split fat sign along with intimate relationship to a nerve trunk help in suggesting the diagnosis.
- Schwannomas are usually located eccentrically in relation to a nerve, whereas neu-rofibromas may be inseparable from the nerve. This differentiation may be difficult to achieve on imaging.
- The distinction between schwannoma and neurofibroma is difficult on imaging though former are expected to show more heterogeneity.
- T2 hyperintense rim and tumoural cysts are more commonly seen in schwannomas.
- Differentiating between malignant and benign neural lesions can be difficult based on imaging alone due to overlapping imaging features in both types.
- Low-flow vascular malformations, myxomas and other soft tissue tumours may mimic nerve sheath tumours on imaging.

SUGGESTED READING

- Assadi, M, Velez, E, Najafi, MH, Matcuk, G, Gholamrezanezhad, A. PET imaging of peripheral nerve tumours. PET Clin. 2019 Jan;14(1):81–89. doi: 10.1016/j.cpet.2018.08.013 Epub 2018 Oct 24. PMID: 30420224.

- Bansal, A, Goyal, S, Goyal, A, Jana, M. WHO classification of soft tissue tumours 2020: An update and simplified approach for radiologists. Eur J Radiol. 2021 Oct;143:109937. doi: 10.1016/j.ejrad.2021.109937. Epub 2021 Aug 28. PMID: 34547634.

- Chee, DW, Peh, WC, Shek, TW. Pictorial essay: Imaging of peripheral nerve sheath tumours. Can Assoc Radiol J. 2011 Aug;62(3):176–182. doi: 10.1016/j.carj.2010.04.009. Epub 2010 May 26. PMID: 20510574.

- Hrehorovich, PA, Franke, HR, Maximin, S, Caracta, P. Malignant peripheral nerve sheath tumour. Radiographics. 2003 May-Jun;23(3):790–794. doi: 10.1148/rg.233025153. PMID: 12740477.

- Kakkar, C, Shetty, CM, Koteshwara, P, Bajpai, S. Telltale signs of peripheral neurogenic tumours on magnetic resonance imaging. Indian J Radiol Imaging. 2015 Oct-Dec;25(4):453–458. doi: 10.4103/0971-3026.169447 PMID: 26752825; PMCID: PMC4693395.

- Lin, J, Martel, W. Cross-sectional imaging of peripheral nerve sheath tumours: Characteristic signs on CT, MR imaging, and sonography. AJR Am J Roentgenol. 2001 Jan;176(1):75–82. doi: 10.2214/ajr.176.1.1760075 PMID: 11133542.

- Pilavaki, M, Chourmouzi, D, Kiziridou, A, Skordalaki, A, Zarampoukas, T, Drevelengas, A. Imaging of peripheral nerve sheath tumours with pathologic correlation: Pictorial review. Eur J Radiol. 2004 Dec;52(3):229–239. doi: 10.1016/j.ejrad.2003.12.001 PMID: 15544900.

- Reynolds, DL Jr, Jacobson, JA, Inampudi, P, Jamadar, DA, Ebrahim, FS, Hayes, CW. Sonographic characteristics of peripheral nerve sheath tumours. Am J Roentgenol. 2004 Mar;182(3):741–744. doi: 10.2214/ajr.182.3.1820741 PMID: 14975979.

- Tagliafico, AS, Isaac, A, Bignotti, B, Rossi, F, Zaottini, F, Martinoli, C. Nerve tumours: What the MSK radiologist should know. Semin Musculoskelet Radiol. 2019 Feb;23(1):76–84. doi: 10.1055/s-0038-1676290 Epub 2019 Jan 30. PMID: 30699454.

- Wilson, MP, Katlariwala, P, Low, G, Murad, MH, McInnes, MDF, Jacques, L, Jack, AS. Diagnostic accuracy of MRI for the detection of malignant peripheral nerve sheath tumours: A systematic review and meta-analysis. AJR Am J Roentgenol. 2021 Jul;217(1):31–39. doi: 10.2214/AJR.20.23403 Epub 2021 Apr 28. PMID: 33909462.

6 Synovial pathologies

Ankita Ahuja,
Nivedita Chakrabarty,
Malini Lawande, Aditya Daftary

INTRODUCTION

Synovial lesions arise from the synovial membrane, a thin specialised mesenchymal soft tissue that outlines the non-articular joint cavity, continuous bursae, recesses and tendinous connections. The synovial membrane also outlines a few bursae separate from the joint cavity, for example, the olecranon bursa. It secretes fluid which provides nutrition and lubrication to the joint cartilage.

WHO classification of soft tissue tumours of 2020 does not categorise synovial tumours and pathologies separately. Pathologically, the synovial lesions can be classified as infectious, inflammatory, deposition-related, degenerative, neoplastic, vascular, non-infectious proliferative disorders and mimics. Radiologically, the lesions can be approached based on their location along the synovium or as intra-articular masses.

Early detection of synovial pathology is essential to prevent intra-articular damage which may lead to osteoarthrosis or irreversible joint damage. Various modalities, including radiographs, ultrasonography and magnetic resonance imaging (MRI), play a role in diagnosing the synovial lesions. Each modality has its challenges, with MRI being the preferred modality.

CLASSIFICATION OF SYNOVIAL LESIONS

Synovial pathologies can be classified into following categories:

1 Infectious
2 Inflammatory
3 Deposition diseases
4 Degenerative
5 Non-infectious proliferative disorders
6 Vascular malformations
7 Neoplastic
8 Mimics: synovial sarcoma, cyclops and synovial cyst.

This chapter will primarily focus on non-infectious proliferative disorders, neoplastic aetiologies, vascular malformations and mimics. The radiological approach is discussed at the end of the chapter.

DOI: 10.1201/9781003218722-6

IMAGING MODALITIES

To address the role of imaging in diagnosing synovial lesions, identify and characterise the following factors:

a   Presence/absence of synovial abnormality by direct visualisation
b   Effects of synovial disease on adjacent bone/soft tissue
c   Imaging characteristics of synovial/intrasynovial contents

Radiographs, computed tomography (CT), ultrasound and MRI independently and in conjunction play a varied role in the diagnostic process.

1 **Radiographs**
   Conventional radiographs are usually the initial imaging modality and may appear normal or demonstrate the indirect effects of synovitis on the soft tissues or bone in the form of joint space widening, periarticular soft tissue swelling, or displaced fat pads and bone erosions, scalloping or remodelling. Calcification or ossification may be identified and their appearance could be diagnostic in certain cases.

2 **Ultrasound**
   Ultrasound is the most easily available imaging modality that directly demonstrates thickened synovium and accompanying joint effusion, especially in superficially placed joints. With the help of Doppler imaging, the vascularity of the lesion can be analysed. Ultrasound may also help identify crystal aggregates in arthropathies with double contour signs in gouty arthritis. Finally, ultrasound guided tissue sampling can be performed.

3 **Computed tomography**
   The osseous effects of synovial pathology can be demonstrated in greater detail by CT, making radiographically occult findings more evident and providing confirmation or better characterisation of suspected or apparent radiographic findings, especially in more complex joints like sacroiliac joints. It also helps identify more subtle calcific/ossific areas within the lesion. Dual-energy CT visualises, characterises and quantifies the monosodium urate crystals in gouty arthritis (see Figure 6.17B).

4 **Magnetic resonance imaging**
   MRI is the most helpful modality for evaluating synovial pathologies. It helps identify thickened synovium, the nature and extent of synovial involvement, as well as assess synovial fluid contents, which play an essential role in the identification and characterisation. It also helps evaluate articular cartilage, subchondral bone, ligaments, muscle and juxta-articular soft tissues, which could be affected as a result of synovitis, and provides valuable clues to the nature of the disease. The signal characteristics of synovium and intrasynovial contents can help in providing a definitive diagnosis. Conventional spin-echo/fast spin-echo T2-weighted (T2W) images should be a part of the imaging protocol to evaluate the signal intensity of the lesion. It is hard to differentiate synovium from effusion on T1-weighted (T1W) images. On fat-suppressed sequences, synovial fluid is hypointense, hyaline cartilage is very bright and the synovium is of intermediate signal intensity. Post-contrast T1-weighted images help differentiate synovium, which enhances from non-enhancing synovial fluid.

● *Non-infectious proliferative synovial lesions*

Pigmented villonodular synovitis

PVNS is characterised by synovial proliferation with hemosiderin pigment deposition which can be intra-articular or extra-articular. Diffuse (more common) and focal are the two forms of intra-articular PVNS. Extra-articular PVNS includes pigmented villonodular bursitis (PVNB) and pigmented villonodular tenosynovitis (PVNTS). It most frequently affects the knee, followed by the hip, ankle and shoulder. It most commonly presents in the second and third decades of life.

Imaging findings

Radiographs may show periarticular soft tissue swelling without calcifications. Bone erosions may be seen in joints having tight capsule such as ankle, hip and elbow. Ultrasound in the diffuse form shows synovial thickening and joint effusion, and in focal form it shows a hypervascular nodule. MRI in diffuse form shows synovial thickening, which is intermediate to hypointense on T1W and hypointense on T2W images due to hemosiderin deposition, and shows blooming on gradient echo (GRE) (Figure 6.1). Inflamed synovium and effusion

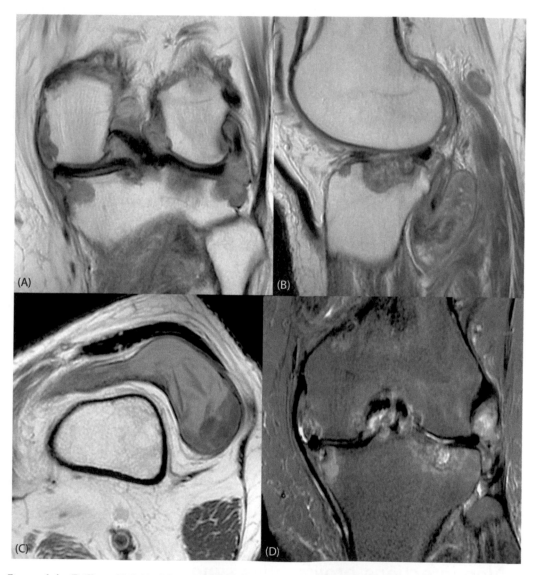

Figure 6.1: Diffuse PVNS: PD weighted (A) coronal, (B) sagittal, (C) axial and (D) fat-suppressed coronal images depicting multiple nodular hypointense lesions in the medial gutter, lateral gutter, suprapatellar recesses, popliteus tendons sheath and intercondylar region with adjoining bone scalloping/erosion and marrow oedema.

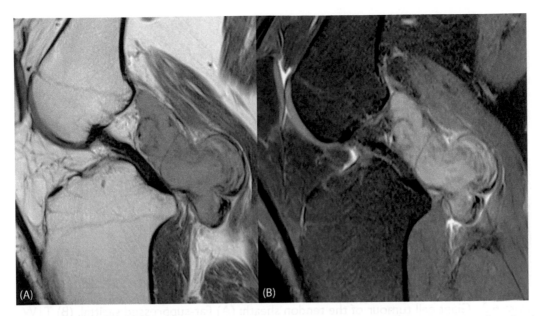

(A) (B)

Figure 6.2: Focal nodular synovitis: (A) PD weighted sagittal and (B) fat-suppressed sagittal images depicting focal nodular hypointense lesion in posterior intercondylar region dorsal to the posterior cruciate ligament.

show T2 hyperintensity. The focal form shows a hypointense nodule on all the sequences (Figure 6.2). These lesions reveal variable post-contrast enhancement.

Giant cell tumour of tendon sheath

As mentioned before, GCTTS is an extra-articular type of PVNS that envelopes the affected tendon. Women in their third to fifth decade of life are most commonly affected. The hand is the most common site of occurrence.

Imaging findings

On a radiograph, a soft tissue mass may be seen with or without adjacent bone erosion/scalloping. Ultrasound shows a well-defined hypervascular lesion closely associated with the tendon sheath. On MRI, a well-defined tumour is seen closely associated with the tendon showing hypointensity on all sequences (Figure 6.3). It shows enhancement on post-contrast scan.

Primary synovial chondromatosis/osteochondromatosis

It is a monoarticular benign process characterised by a chondroid metaplastic change in the synovium. It is more common in men in their third to fifth decades of life. It preferentially affects large joints, with knee being the most frequently involved site. There are three phases of the disease: the initial phase, transitional phase and an inactive phase. In the initial phase, there is formation of cartilaginous masses due to metaplastic change within the synovium; free bodies are formed in the transitional phase due to detached cartilaginous nodules; and in the inactive phase, there is resolution of the synovial proliferation with the presence of uniform-sized loose bodies and variable joint effusion. Majority (70–90%) of the cartilaginous nodules undergo calcification and even ossification.

Imaging findings

Imaging varies depending on the phase of disease. Radiographs may be unremarkable in the initial phases with no mineralisation of the bodies but later with mineralisation may reveal uniform-sized calcified/ossified free bodies (Figure 6.4). Ring- and arc-like pattern of chondral calcifications may be seen. Ultrasound shows heterogeneous mass with hyperechoic

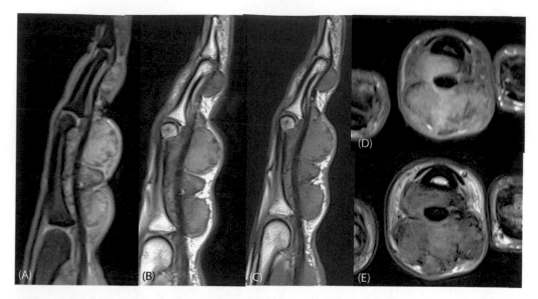

Figure 6.3: Giant cell tumour of the tendon sheath: (A) Fat-suppressed sagittal, (B) T1W sagittal, (C) T2W sagittal, (D) fat-suppressed axial and (E) T2W axial images demonstrate hypointense nodular lesions surrounding the flexor tendon of the finger at proximal and middle phalanx levels.

foci suggestive of chondroid bodies which are hypovascular on Doppler. Osseous bodies show posterior acoustic shadowing. CT better depicts the ossified masses. MRI appearance depends on the stage of the disease. In the initial stage, intrasynovial cartilaginous masses show intermediate signal on T1W and hyperintense signal on T2W images without areas of internal signal void with intense post-contrast enhancement (Figure 6.5A). Post-contrast

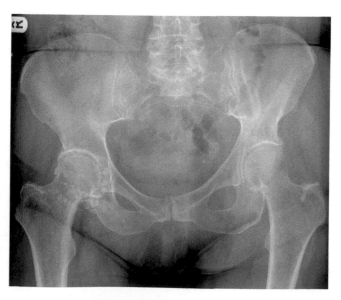

Figure 6.4: Primary synovial osteochondromatosis: Anteroposterior radiograph of the pelvis depicting numerous rounded osseous bodies within the right hip joint. Please appreciate preserved hip joint space contrary to the secondary osteochondromatosis which shows underlying joint space reduction and other findings of osteoarthritis. (Image Credits: Dr. Harun Gupta, Leeds Teaching Hospitals NHS Trust, Leeds, UK.)

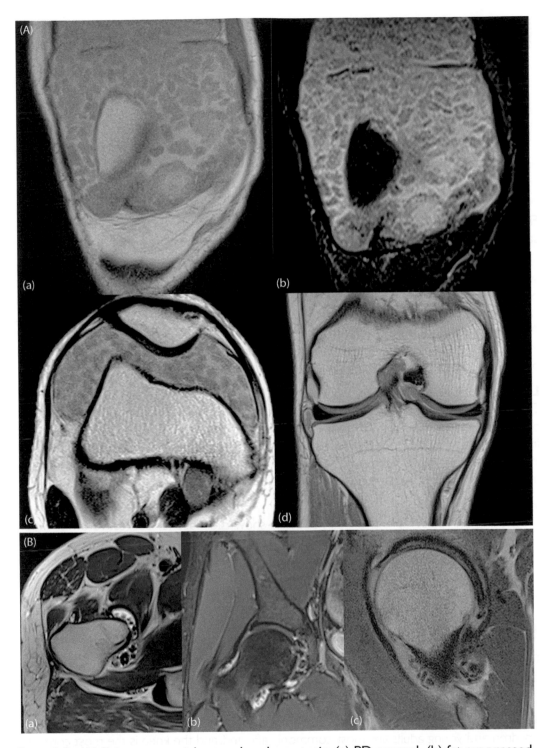

Figure 6.5: (A) Primary synovial osteochondromatosis: (a) PD coronal, (b) fat-suppressed coronal, (c) PD axial depicts multiple similar sized intermediate intensity *cartilaginous* intra-articular bodies and (d) PD coronal depicts intact articular cartilage. (B) Primary synovial osteochondromatosis: (a) T2 axial, (b) fat-suppressed coronal and (c) PD sagittal images depict multiple similar sized hypointense *calcified* intra-articular bodies with relatively intact articular cartilage.

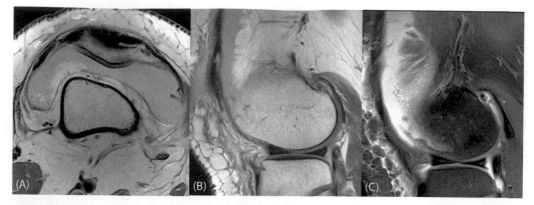

Figure 6.6: Lipoma arborescens: (A) PD axial, (B) PD sagittal and (C) fat-suppressed sagittal images depict focal fatty nodular synovial lesion in the lateral suprapatellar recess.

scan can differentiate uncalcified masses from synovial fluid. In the second phase, the synovial bodies are T2 hyperintense, T1 low to intermediate intensity with central signal void from calcification or central fat and a low signal rim depending on mineralisation (Figure 6.5B). Areas of low signal are seen within the calcified intrasynovial cartilaginous nodules. Calcified free bodies are hypointense on all the pulse sequences. Ossified nodules show low signal peripheral cortical bone and high signal central fatty marrow.

Lipoma arborescens

There is villous lipomatous benign proliferation of the synovial tissue in this disorder. It occurs more commonly in men in their fifth to sixth decades of life. The knee is the most frequent site. It is considered to be a non-specific reactive response to chronic synovial irritation rather than a neoplasm. There may be an association with osteoarthritis, rheumatoid arthritis or trauma in certain cases.

Imaging findings

Diagnosing on radiographs is difficult but may show radiolucency suggestive of fat within areas of increased density within the synovial pouch or articular recess. MRI may show subsynovial mass-like fat deposits (Figure 6.6) or frond-like fat intensity areas projecting inward from the synovium (Figure 6.7). The large joint effusion may be seen and chemical shift artefacts may be seen at the interface of synovial lesion and effusion.

● *Vascular malformations*

These are classified as capillary, venous, arterial, lymphatic or mixed types. They are congenital and increase slowly, presenting during childhood or adolescence. The knee is the most commonly affected joint.

Synovial haemangioma

Children and young adults are most commonly affected, and the knee is the most common location.

Imaging findings

Radiographs may show non-specific soft tissue swelling with or without phleboliths and associated osteopenia. Ultrasound also helps localise the lesion with vascularity demonstrated on Doppler images (Figure 6.8). MRI shows intra-articular lobulated mass without mass effect. It is T1 intermediate with intralesional fat showing areas of hyperintensity, T2 hyperintense

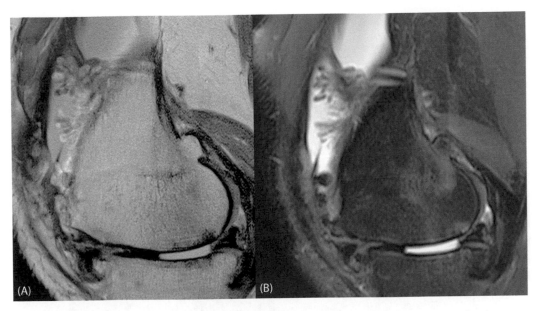

Figure 6.7: Lipoma arborescens: (A) PD sagittal and (B) fat-suppressed sagittal images depict focal frond-like fat intensity area projecting inward from the synovium in the medial suprapatellar recess.

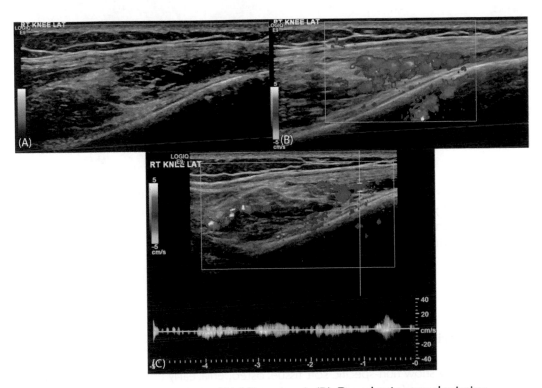

Figure 6.8: Synovial haemangioma: (A) Ultrasound, (B) Doppler images depicting multiple anechoic vascular channels with colour flow, and (C) spectral waveforms within the lesion. (Image Courtesy of Dr. Harun Gupta.)

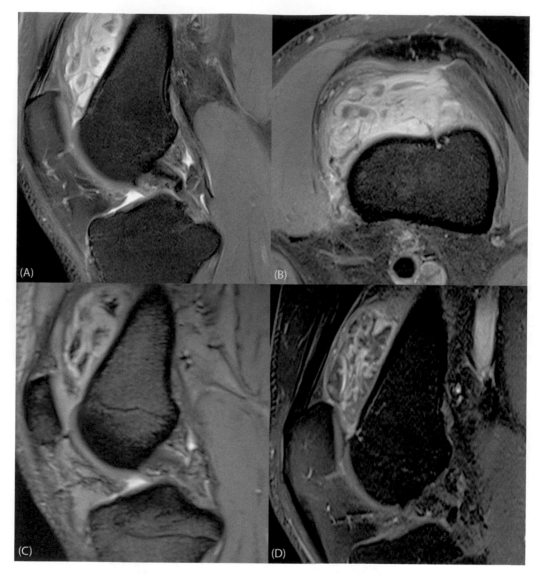

Figure 6.9: Synovial haemangioma: (A) PD fat-suppressed sagittal and (B) axial images depicting STIR hyperintense suprapatellar lesion with voids which on (C) gradient-echo images are blooming suggesting calcification and (D) post-contrast images reveal intense enhancement with non-enhancing calcific areas.

with hypointense septae within and reveals intense heterogeneous enhancement. Phleboliths can be identified (Figure 6.9). Pressure erosions of bones can occur if there is extra-articular involvement.

Synovial arteriovenous malformation

Imaging findings

Radiographs may show non-specific soft tissue, osteopenia, early epiphyseal maturation, leg length discrepancy or features of arthropathy. Ultrasound shows a heterogeneous lesion with vascular channels. On MRI, synovial arteriovenous vascular malformations reveal high-flow serpentine vascular channels seen as flow voids without well-defined mass. The post-contrast scan helps evaluate feeding arteries and draining veins.

● *Neoplastic pathologies*

Synovial chondrosarcoma

It is a very rare neoplasm. It can either be a primary lesion or secondary to synovial chondromatosis, later being more common. The relative risk of progression of synovial chondromatosis to malignancy is reported to be 5%. This occurs due to the metaplastic transformation of the synovium. Several cartilaginous nodules may form which may or may not calcify or ossify. It most commonly occurs in the fourth to seventh decades of life, with knee and hip being the most common sites.

Imaging findings

Radiographs show soft tissue masses within the joints which may show calcified bodies. Imaging features are similar to chondromatosis. On MRI, synovial chondrosarcoma appears as a lobulated mass showing a hyperintense signal on T2W image. Calcification within the nodule shows a hypointense signal on all the sequences. Extension into the adjacent soft tissues and extrinsic erosion of bone suggest an aggressive process, but maybe seen in both conditions. Metastasis is indicative of malignancy.

Synovial metastasis

It is rare for the malignant disease to spread to the synovium. Primary lung cancer is the most common tumour to metastasise to the synovium and the knee is the most common site. It has a poor prognosis with survival of less than five months.

● *Mimics*

Synovial sarcoma

It arises from primitive mesenchymal cells in the extra-articular soft tissues and not from the synovium. It is named so because of its similarity to synovial tissue at light microscopy.

Synovial sarcoma comprises 10% of all the primary malignant soft tissue tumours. It most commonly presents in young adults. Tumours sized >5 cm have a poor prognosis. The popliteal fossa is the most common location and 5% of cases can present within the joints.

Imaging findings

Radiographs may show calcified masses in 20 to 30% of the cases. Ultrasound shows a hypoechoic lesion. CT shows a necrotic, haemorrhagic or calcified mass. Calcifications can be punctate or peripheral. MRI best depicts these lesions, which are situated close to bones. It is hypointense on T1W image and heterogeneous on T2W image, containing hypointense signal due to calcification/fibrosis, isointense solid components, and hyperintense haemorrhagic or necrotic areas comprising the triple sign (Figure 6.10). This lesion shows enhancement in the arterial phase. PET-CT shows a high standardised uptake value.

Synovial cyst

A synovial cyst is herniation of the synovial membrane through the joint capsule and contains synovial fluid. They can occur in every joint and also around the tendon sheath and bursae. Baker's cyst or popliteal cyst is the most characteristic example representing the distention of a pre-existing medial gastrocnemius-semimembranosus bursa in the popliteal fossa. On MRI, it is hypointense on T1W and hyperintense on T2W images (Figure 6.11).

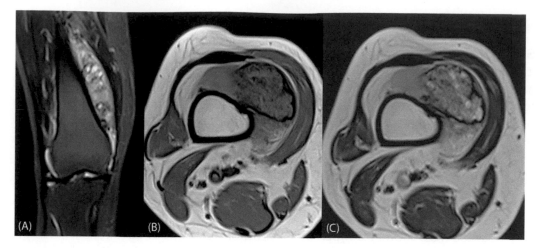

Figure 6.10: Synovial sarcoma: (A) TIW, (B) T2W and (C) post-contrast axial images depicting lesion in the distal leg with iso- to hypointense on TIW, predominantly intermediate intensity on T2W images with central hyperintensity (necrosis) and intensely enhancing on post-contrast images.

Cyclops lesion

Cyclops lesion is localised anterior arthrofibrosis, a complication of anterior cruciate ligament reconstruction surgery. The exact aetiology is unknown; it may be related to gradual fraying of the graft or uplifting of fibrocartilaginous tissue during tibial tunnel drilling. On MRI, a soft tissue mass is seen in the anterior intercondylar notch near the tibial tunnel of the anterior cruciate ligament graft (Figure 6.12). Due to the fibrous content, it is of intermediate to low signal intensity on all pulse sequences.

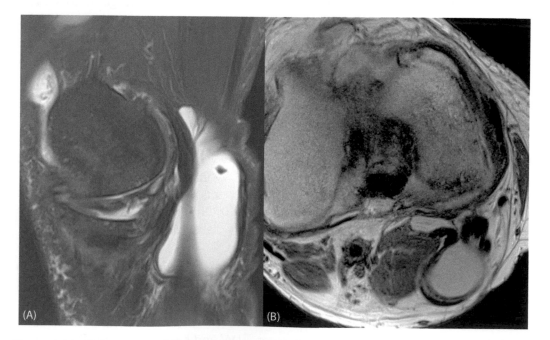

Figure 6.11: Baker's cyst: (A) Fat-suppressed sagittal and (B) PD axial images depicting medial gastrocnemius-semimembranosus bursa in the popliteal fossa.

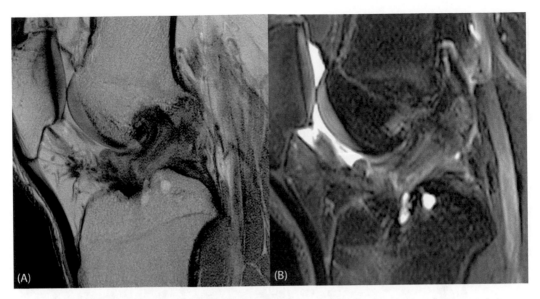

Figure 6.12: Cyclops: (A) PD and (B) fat-suppressed sagittal images depicting nodule formation in the anterior intercondylar region near the tibial tunnel of the anterior cruciate ligament graft.

● *Infectious pathologies*

Septic arthritis is a common disease entity. Joint effusion is considered the most common finding. Synovial thickening is also appreciated in a small percentage of cases. Ultrasound and MRI help detect synovial thickening. Ultrasound can be used for performing guided tissue sampling. MRI also helps evaluate the bone marrow, soft tissues and joints (Figure 6.13). Delay in diagnosis may lead to complications such as secondary osteoarthritis, osteomyelitis, etc.

● *Inflammatory diseases*

Rheumatoid arthritis
Rheumatoid arthritis is a chronic, progressively destructive systemic inflammatory disease affecting synovial joints. Pannus represents a proliferative hyperplastic, hypervascular locally invasive synovial reaction leading to irreversible joint damage. The fibrous pannus represents the end stage of this synovial proliferation. Women are more commonly affected between fourth and sixth decade of life. The most frequently affected joints are hands, wrists and feet.

Imaging findings
In the end stages, radiographs show soft tissue swelling, marginal erosions, periarticular osteopenia, joint space narrowing and joint subluxation. Ultrasound and MRI detect synovial proliferation (Figure 6.14), tenosynovitis and bone erosions. Pannus is intermediate to low signal intensity soft tissue on T1W and T2W images (Figure 6.15). Compared to chronic infective arthritis (tuberculosis), the synovium in rheumatoid arthritis is thick and bulky with more frequent bone erosions.

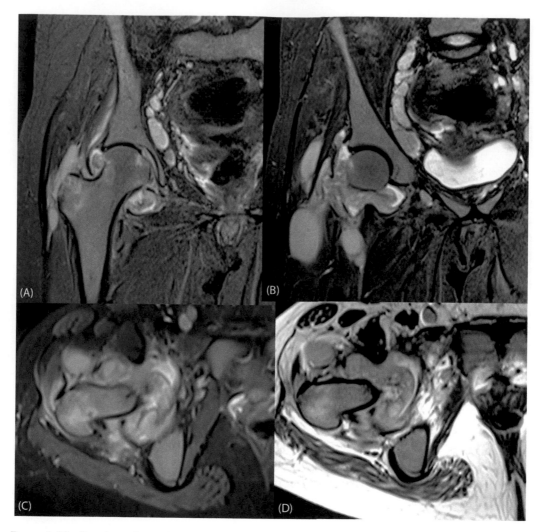

Figure 6.13: Septic arthritis hip: (A), (B) Fat-suppressed coronals, (C) axial and (D) PD axial images depict intermediate intensity synovial thickening with hyperintense joint effusion, adjoining marrow oedema with enlarged iliac lymph nodes.

Gouty arthritis

Gout is a hyperuricemic metabolic disorder with resultant deposition of sodium monourate crystals within or around the joints. Tophi represent a chronic phase of gout in which there are local aggregates of urate crystals and a proteinaceous matrix surrounded by an intense inflammatory response. It usually presents as asymmetric polyarthritis. Men are more frequently affected in their fifth to seventh decades of life. The most common locations for tophi are hands and feet joints.

Imaging findings

On radiographs, chronic tophaceous gout reveals juxta-articular soft tissue masses with sharply defined erosions (Figure 6.16) and overhanging margins of bone. Tophi on MRI reveal T2 variable signal intensity with heterogeneous intermediate to low signal intensity patterns being the most common, likely due to the presence of urate crystals and fibrous tissue

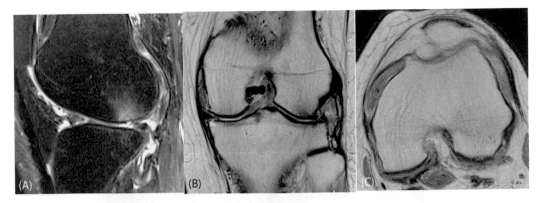

Figure 6.14: Rheumatoid arthritis knee: A young female patient with (A) fat-suppressed sagittal, (B) PD coronal and (C) axial images depicts medial and lateral osteoarthrosis with synovial thickening in the gutters.

(Figure 6.17A). Post-contrast images reveal intense enhancement reflecting the increased inflammatory response. DECT acts as a problem-solving tool which can depict infiltrating monosodium urate crystals in classical anatomical sites (Figure 6.17B).

● *Deposition diseases*

Amyloid arthropathy
Amyloid arthropathy affects joints bilaterally with an accumulation of amyloids in and around the joints. The most frequently affected joints are the shoulders, hips, knees and wrists.

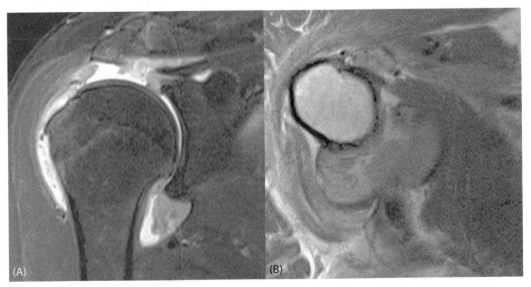

Figure 6.15: Rheumatoid arthritis shoulder: A young female patient with (A) fat-suppressed coronal and (B) PD axial images depicting supraspinatus full-thickness tear with joint effusion and extensive synovial thickening; most prominent in the inferior axillary recess.

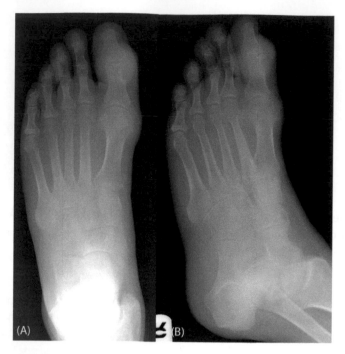

Figure 6.16: Gouty arthropathy: (A) Frontal and (B) oblique radiographs of the foot reveal soft tissue swelling along the first distal interphalangeal joint with erosion along the medial margin of the proximal phalanx.

Imaging findings

Conventional radiographs and CT scans include juxta-articular soft tissue masses, peri-articular osteopenia, subchondral cysts, joint effusions and erosions. The joint spaces are preserved. MRI reveals low to intermediate signal intensity amyloid deposits on all pulse sequences (Figure 6.18).

● *Degenerative diseases*

Secondary synovial chondromatosis/osteochondromatosis

It is seen in association with trauma, osteoarthritis or inflammatory arthritis. Knee, hip and shoulder are the joints most commonly affected.

Imaging findings

The radiograph shows a few varying-sized intra-articular loose bodies showing multiple rings of calcification. Underlying degenerative changes are seen within the joints. CT can depict these calcified loose bodies and extrinsic bone erosions. MRI may show hypointense loose bodies on GRE. T1W and T2W images may show these loose bodies with fatty marrow and hypointense cortex.

RADIOLOGICAL APPROACH TO SYNOVIAL LESIONS

Each modality plays its role in diagnosing the synovial pathologies, of which MRI is the pre-ferred modality. As discussed in the chapter, radiologic anatomic knowledge of the synovial

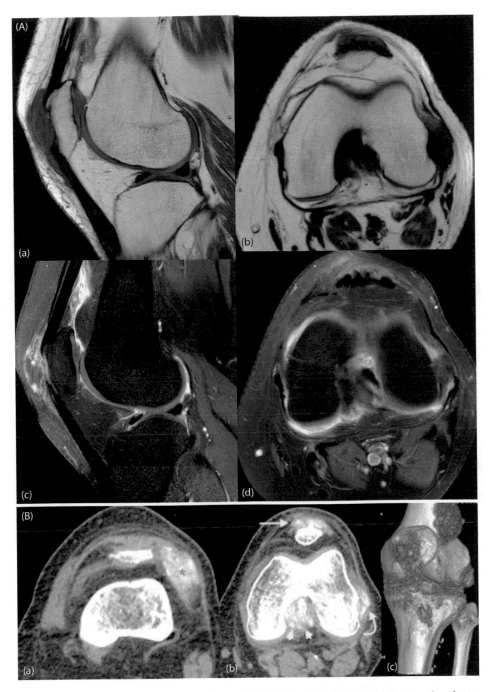

Figure 6.17: (A) Gouty arthropathy: (a) Sagittal T1, (b) axial T2W images reveal soft tissue along the patellar tendon and popliteal tendon origins with peripheral enhancement on post-contrast (c) sagittal and (d) axial images. (Image Credits: Dr Harun Gupta, Leeds Teaching Hospitals NHS Trust, Leeds, UK). (B) DECT in gout: Axial CT images of the same patient in soft tissue window at the level of suprapatellar pouch (a) and the popliteal groove (b) showing soft tissue and superimposed calcium deposits in the vastus lateralis (red asterisk), patellar tendon (long yellow arrow), PCL (yellow arrowheads) and popliteal tendon (curved arrow), and corresponding volume-reconstructed DECT image (c) demonstrating extensive monosodium urate crystal deposition within the knee (violet colour-coded). (Image Credits: Dr Harun Gupta, Leeds Teaching Hospitals NHS Trust, Leeds, UK.)

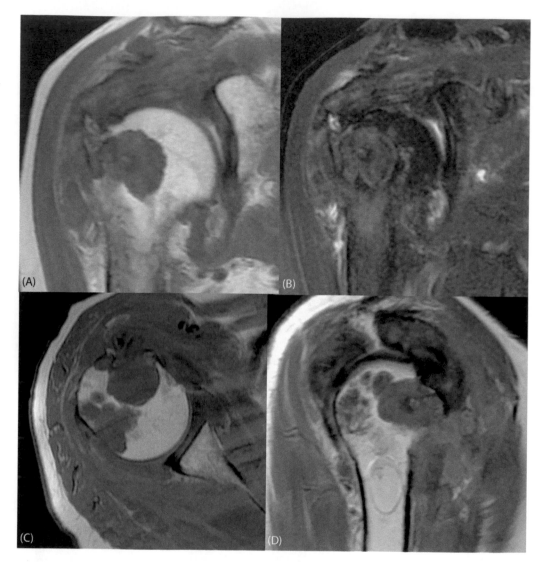

Figure 6.18: Amyloid arthropathy: PD Coronal (A) fat-suppressed coronal (B), PD axial (C) and sagittal (D) images depicting large hypointense deposits, also extending along the rotator cuff tendons and causing bone erosions.

lining with characteristic imaging appearances helps to narrow down the differential diagnosis and even make a confident diagnosis.

On MRI, the first step is to determine if the lesion is seen extending along the synovium (smooth and diffuse vs. nodular) or presenting as an intra-articular lesion (focal vs. multiple), as discussed in Table 6.1. Further, the lesions can be characterised based on their T2 signal intensity, associated bone changes (scalloping/erosion), associated calcification/haemorrhage and enhancement pattern, as depicted in Table 6.2.

Table 6.1: Radiological Approach to Synovial Lesions

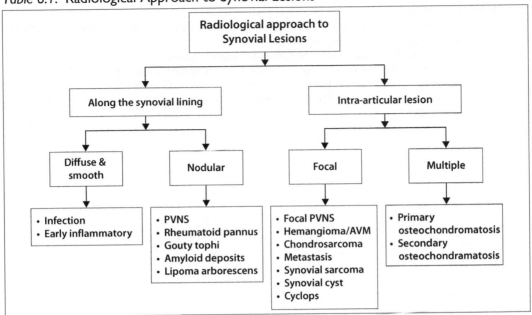

Table 6.2: Characterisation of Synovial Lesions

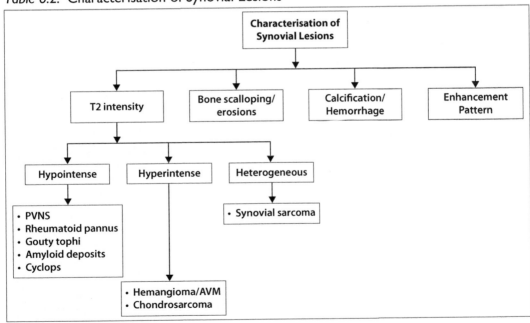

SUGGESTED READING

- Karchevsky, M, Schweitzer, ME, Morrison, WB, Parellada, JA. MRI findings of septic arthritis and associated osteomyelitis in adults. Am J Roentgenol. 2004 Jan;182(1):119–122.
- Mohey, N, Hassan, TA. Feasibility of MRI in diagnosis and characterization of intra-articular synovial masses and mass-like lesions. Egypt J Radiol Nucl Med. 2020 Dec;51(1):1–1.
- Murphey, MD, Rhee, JH, Lewis, RB, Fanburg-Smith, JC, Flemming, DJ, Walker, EA. Pigmented villonodular synovitis: Radiologic-pathologic correlation. Radiographics. 2008 Sep;28(5):1493–1518.

- Murphey, MD, Vidal, JA, Fanburg-Smith, JC, Gajewski, DA. Imaging of synovial chondromatosis with radiologic-pathologic correlation. Radiographics. 2007;27(5):1465–1488.
- Narváez, JA, Narváez, J, Aguilera, C, De Lama, E, Portabella, F. MR imaging of synovial tumors and tumor-like lesions. Eur. Radiol. 2001 Dec;11(12):2549–2560.
- Narváez, JA, Narváez, J, Ortega, R, De Lama, E, Roca, Y, Vidal, N. Hypointense synovial lesions on T2-weighted images: Differential diagnosis with pathologic correlation. Am J Roentgenol. 2003 Sep;181(3):761–769.
- Sheldon, PJ, Forrester, DM, Learch, TJ. Imaging of intraarticular masses. Radiographics. 2005 Jan;25(1):105–119.
- Turan, A, Çeltikçi, P, Tufan, A, Öztürk, MA. Basic radiological assessment of synovial diseases: A pictorial essay. Eur J Rheumatol. 2017 Jun;4(2):166.

Muscle tumours

Hayder Al-Assam,
Ganesh Hegde, Rajesh Botchu

INTRODUCTION

The tumours of muscular origin are relatively uncommon, accounting for only 2% of all soft tissue tumours and about 10% of malignant soft tissue tumours. They can be divided histologically into smooth muscle tumours and skeletal muscle tumours according to the type of muscle cells. There are also number of miscellaneous intramuscular tumours which originate from intramuscular remanent tissues such as intramuscular lipoma and myxoma. This chapter aims to give an overview of the muscle tissue tumours and their radiological features. The chapter also provides an experienced view of the diagnostic pathways to reach a final diagnosis of such tumours.

CURRENT APPROACH TO MUSCLE TUMOUR DIAGNOSIS

Like with other soft tissue lesions, ultrasound is the modality of choice for initial evaluation and guidance if a biopsy is contemplated, particularly if tumour is located superficially. Computed tomography (CT) may be useful in evaluation if the location of the lesion is in the head and neck or in retroperitoneum. Apart from visualising the extent and infiltration of the primary lesion, it is used to exclude distant metastasis.

Magnetic resonance imaging (MRI) is the preferred modality for evaluating these lesions due to its ability to accurately depict the location, extent, internal content and relationship with surrounding structures, thus providing valuable information for planning further steps such as tissue sampling and surgery. Although there have been modifications to the skeletal muscle tumour category based on advances in genetic mutations, advanced MRI sequences have not provided similar insight into the tumour category. There are no diagnostic imaging features that enable diagnostic certainty without a biopsy.

WHO CLASSIFICATION

According to the recent update of the World Health Organization classification of soft tissue tumours, the tumours of muscular origin can be divided into:

1 Tumours of skeletal muscle origin
   a Benign primary tumours which include rhabdomyomas.
   b Malignant primary tumours include rhabdomyosarcoma and ectomesenchymoma. The rhabdomyosarcomas can be subdivided into embryonal, alveolar, pleomorphic and spindle cell types.

DOI: 10.1201/9781003218722-7

2 Tumours of smooth muscle origin

   a Benign tumours include leiomyoma.

   b Malignant tumours are leiomyosarcoma and inflammatory leiomyosarcoma.

We have described intramuscular myxoma (Chapter 9) and intramuscular haemangioma (chapter 8) separately as they are rather "located" in the muscles than "primarily originated" from the muscle tissue.

● *Adult rhabdomyoma*

Adult rhabdomyomas are rare benign tumours of the skeletal muscles. They are the most common subtype of the extra-cardiac rhabdomyoma. It is worth noting that malignant rhabdomyosarcoma is more common than benign rhabdomyoma. Adult rhabdomyoma arises in patients over 40 years of age in 3 to 5 males compared to 1 female. They most commonly occur in head and neck region as solitary masses but can also be multifocal in approximately 15% of cases.

Other types of rhabdomyomas include fetal rhabdomyoma which occurs mainly in males in the head and neck region at birth. Genital rhabdomyoma occurs in the vagina and vulva of middle-aged females. These two subtypes are exceedingly rare compared to adult form.

MRI usually shows a well-defined homogenous mass with slight high signal intensity on T1 and T2 compared to adjacent muscles and with mild contrast enhancement. On CT scans, they appear as well-defined homogenous enhancing mass. On ultrasound, they appear as well-circumscribed homogenous low echoic masses.

● *Rhabdomyosarcoma*

This is the malignant form of skeletal muscle tumour. This is also most common in children and accounts for 19% of all paediatric soft tissue malignant sarcomas and about 5 to 8% of childhood cancer. The age at the diagnosis is generally below 45 years with about 65% diagnosed under the age of 10 years. In contrast to rhabdomyoma, the rhabdomyosarcomas are mostly sporadic cases but may be seen with other congenital anomalies such as neurofibromatosis type 1 (NF1), Beckwith–Wiedemann syndrome, Li-Fraumeni syndrome, DICER1 syndrome, Costello syndrome and maternal use of cocaine and marijuana.

Clinical presentation depends on the location (biliary tract, genitourinary, heart, head and neck or in the orbit); however, they are generally rapidly growing tumours causing local mass effect on the adjacent neurovascular bundles and have tendencies to infiltrate adjacent bones and may lead to pathological fractures. They occur predominantly in the region of head, neck and pelvis in children.

Histologically these can be divided into three types:
1 Embryonal rhabdomyosarcoma
   ● Spindle cell rhabdomyosarcoma: 50 to 66%
   ● Botryoid rhabdomyosarcoma: 5 to 10% (best prognosis)
   ● Anaplastic rhabdomyosarcoma
2 Alveolar rhabdomyosarcoma: 20%
3 Pleomorphic rhabdomyosarcoma: 5%

The embryonal rhabdomyosarcoma is the most common subtype of rhabdomyosarcoma, representing about 50 to 70% of all cases. They can also be subdivided into spindle cell rhabdomyosarcoma, botryoid rhabdomyosarcoma and anaplastic rhabdomyosarcoma. These are typically seen in children below the age of 15 years. They are generally homogenous and when located in limbs can lead to bowing of the long bones of the extremities in children.

The alveolar rhabdomyosarcomas account for 20 to 40% of all rhabdomyosarcomas, which can be located anywhere in the body, more frequently in the deep compartment of the extremities. This subtype has the worst prognosis.

The pleomorphic rhabdomyosarcoma is the least common subtype (only 5%) that tends to occur in adults over the age of 40 years and is sometimes difficult to distinguish from other pleomorphic sarcomas such as malignant fibrous histiocytoma. They follow the general non-specific appearance of the rhabdomyosarcoma but it may contain areas of necrosis.

Radiological features of the rhabdomyosarcomas are non-specific on plain films, but may show calcifications, bony involvement and sometimes metastases. The mass itself appears as soft tissue density, and it when occurs in the limbs of a child, embryonal rhabdomyosarcoma may result in bowing of the adjacent long bones. This should not be mistaken for slow-growing tumours of benign nature.

Under ultrasound they appear as heterogenous well-defined mass with irregular margins and low to medium echogenicity. CT scan shows soft tissue enhancing mass (Figure 7.1) and adjacent bone destruction in over one-fifth of the cases.

MRI features are more variable, especially between subtypes (Figures 7.2 and 7.3). In T1-weighted images, they appear as low to intermediate T1 signal compared to adjacent muscle with areas of haemorrhages and necrosis, especially common in alveolar and pleomorphic subgroups and mostly homogenous in embryonal subtype. On T2-weighted images, they are high T2 signal masses with flow voids. Contrast enhancement is marked with gadolinium. The embryonal subtype is associated with ring-like enhancement.

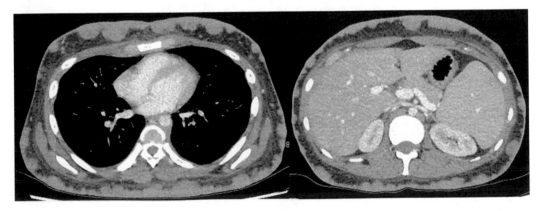

Figure 7.1: **Metastatic rhadomyosarcoma: Contrast-enhanced axial CT images, above (A) and below (B) the level of the diaphragm, show extensive subdermal infiltration by enhancing mass lesions in a histopathologically proven case of metastatic rhabdomyosarcoma. (Image Courtesy of Dr. Harun Gupta.)**

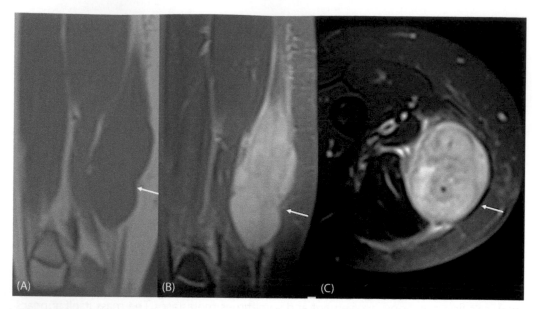

Figure 7.2: Rhabdomyosarcoma in an adolescent. Coronal T1-weighted (A), STIR (B) and axial T2-weighted fat-suppressed (C) images showing a large tumour (arrow) within the posterior muscle compartment of the thigh. There is significant mass effect and perilesional extracapsular oedema tracking along the fascial planes consistent with aggressive nature of the lesion. Unfused distal femoral physes are also visible on coronal images.

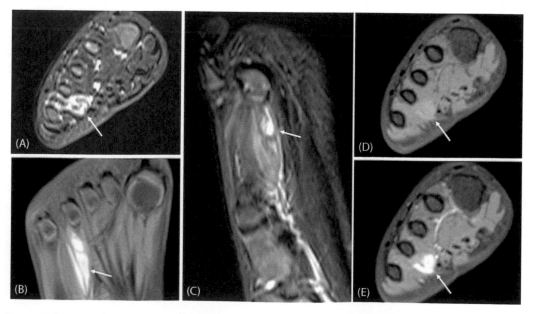

Figure 7.3: Rhabdomyosarcoma alveolar. Coronal STIR (A), axial T2-weighted fat-suppressed (B), STIR sagittal (C), T1-weighted fat-suppressed coronal pre- (D) and post-contrast (E) images showing enhancing lesion in the plantar aspect of the foot (arrow). Imaging appearances are non-specific and it is impossible diagnose rhabdomyosarcoma on the basis of imaging alone.

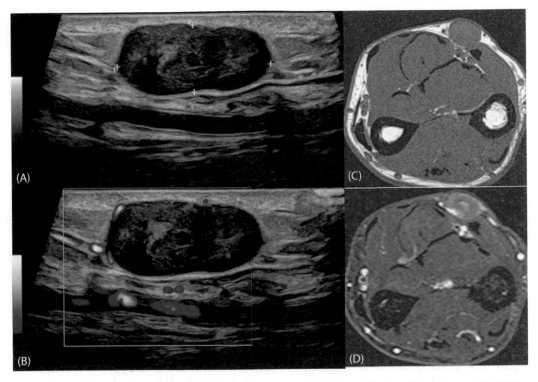

Figure 7.4: Leiomyoma. Greyscale (A) and colour Doppler (B) ultrasound images depict a forearm soft tissue mass overlying the ulnar neurovascular bundle and corresponding TI-weighted (C) and STIR (D) axial images through the mid-forearm level show a non-specific encapsulated mass lesion overlying the ulnar neurovascular bundle which proved to be a leiomyoma on histopathology. (Image Courtesy of Dr. Harun Gupta.)

● *Leiomyoma*

It is a benign tumour of the smooth muscle cells. The most common locations are uterine, cervical, urinary tract, urethral, vascular (angioleiomyoma) oesophageal and small intestine. Due to the nature of this chapter and its focus on soft tissue pathologies, only brief description of features is included in this chapter. Soft tissue leiomyomas are extremely rare and they are diagnosis of exclusion, generally diagnosed only on histopathology (Figure 7.4). The malignant variant of this smooth muscle tumour is called leiomyosarcoma.

● *Leiomyosarcomas*

Leiomyosarcomas are rare malignant variants of the smooth muscle tumours, accounting for about 8% of malignant soft tissue tumours. Similar to their benign variant, they can occur in any organ (Figure 7.5) with smooth muscles in their structure. They tend to become larger masses before diagnosis especially in the abdominal and pelvic cavities. They have a variable appearance of ultrasound. On CT scan, they are generally heterogeneous masses with central necrosis but no calcification which occurs in benign lesion more frequently. On MRI, they appear isointense on TI, intermediate or hyperintense to fat on T2 and mainly hyperintense on T2 fat-saturated sequences (Figure 7.6).

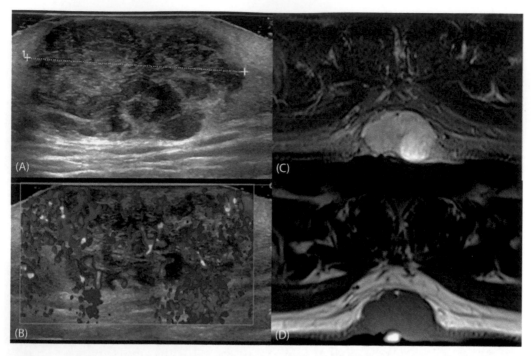

Figure 7.5: Leiomyosarcoma, grade II. Greyscale (A) and colour Doppler (B) images demonstrate a large complex soft tissue mass lesion in the lower back midline showing disorganised internal vascularity. STIR (C) and T1-weighted (D) axial images show corresponding aggressive appearing superficial soft tissue mass which on biopsy proved to be grade II leiomyosarcoma. (Image Courtesy of Dr. Harun Gupta.)

● *Skeletal muscle metastasis*

Skeletal muscle metastases are uncommon, accounting for 0.03% to 17% and are seen in widespread disease or post-mortem studies. The most common primary cancer is lung carcinoma, but others could include pancreatic, renal, colorectal, gastric, ovarian, oesophageal cancers and malignant melanoma. The most common location for metastasis is

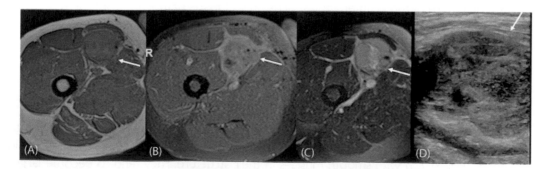

Figure 7.6: Leiomyosarcoma. Axial T1-weighted (A), STIR (B), T1-weighted fat-suppressed post-contrast (C) and greyscale ultrasound (D) images show a large deep-seated heterogenous soft tissue mass encasing the femoral neurovascular bundle (arrow) which appears isointense on T1-weighted images and markedly heterogeneous on STIR and post-gadolinium images.

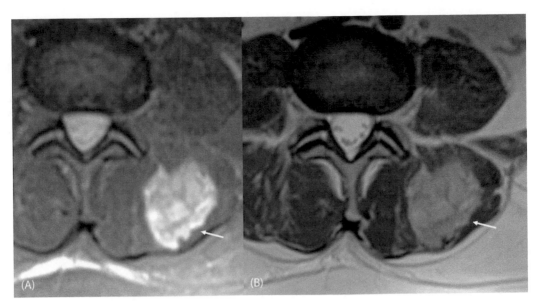

Figure 7.7: Skeletal muscle metastasis. Axial STIR (A) and T2-weighted (B) images showing intramuscular metastasis in the left paraspinal muscles.

iliopsoas muscle followed by gluteal, paraspinal, lower limb, abdominal wall and thoracic wall muscles.

Radiological features in CT show intramuscular hypodense lesion with peripheral enhancement. In MRI, the lesion shows a low signal on T1, a heterogenous signal on T2 with perilesional oedema and peripheral enhancement with contrast. (Figure 7.7) Ultrasound features are variable but generally heterogenous echogenicity lesions in the muscles.

Take-home points

1 Tumours of muscular origin are uncommon and WHO classifies them mainly as smooth and skeletal muscle tumours.
2 Ultrasound and MRI are preferred for local staging when the lesion is superficial. CT is useful when the lesion is located in the head and neck, abdomen or retroperitoneum and also for evaluation of the distant metastasis.
3 Although some of the lesions of muscle origin can be diagnosed based on imaging, majority of them require histopathology for definitive diagnosis.

SUGGESTED READING

- Ahlawat, S, M. Fayad, L. Revisiting the WHO classification system of soft tissue tumours: Emphasis on advanced magnetic resonance imaging sequences. Part 1. Pol J Radiol. 2020;85(1):396–408.
- Damjanov, I. Enzinger and Weiss's soft tissue tumors, 5th edition. Shock. 2008;30(6):754.
- de Trey, L, Schmid, S, Huber, G Multifocal adult rhabdomyoma of the head and neck manifestation in 7 locations and review of the literature. Case Report Otolaryngol. 2013;2013:1–5.
- Evans, JC, Curtis, J. The radiological appearances of tuberous sclerosis. Br J Radiol. 2000;73(865):91–98.
- Grebenc, ML, Rosado de christenson, ML, Burke, AP et al. Primary cardiac and pericardial neoplasms: Radiologic-pathologic correlation. Radiographics. 2000;20(4):1073–103.
- Kransdorf, M, Murphey, M. Imaging of soft tissue tumors. Philadelphia: Lippincott Williams & Wilkins; 2006.

- Petscavage-Thomas, J, Walker, E, Logie, C, Clarke, L, Duryea, D, Murphey, M. Soft-tissue myxomatous lesions: Review of salient imaging features with pathologic comparison. Radiographics. 2014;34(4):964–980.
- Schepper, A. Imaging of soft tissue tumors. Berlin: Springer; 2006.
- Surov, A, Hainz, M, Holzhausen, H, Arnold, D, Katzer, M, Schmidt, J, Spielmann, R, Behrmann, C. Skeletal muscle metastases: Primary tumours, prevalence, and radiological features. Eur Radiol. 2009;20(3):649–658.
- Weinreb, J, Barkoff, N, Megibow, A, Demopoulos, R. The value of MR imaging in distinguishing leiomyomas from other solid pelvic masses when sonography is indeterminate. Am J Roentgenol. 1990;154(2):295–299.

8 Vascular tumours

Ajay Maliyakkal

INTRODUCTION

Vascular tumours arise from the proliferation of endothelial cells. The spectrum ranges from haemangioma in the benign category, Kaposiform and other haemangioendotheliomas and Kaposi's sarcoma in the intermediate category to angiosarcoma and epithelioid haemangioendothelioma in the malignant group.

Benign vascular tumours can be found in any organ and can involve multiple organs as part of an angiomatous syndrome. Vascular invasion by tumour is a multisystem phenomenon with major prognostic implications.

Imaging plays a critical role in determination of benign versus malignant nature and delineation of tumour extent. In addition, knowledge of tumour location and typical features can facilitate accurate diagnosis.

In this chapter, we look at the common ultrasound, computed tomography (CT) and magnetic resonance imaging (MRI) findings on selected benign and malignant primary vascular tumours and identify tumour-like conditions at the end the chapter.

Apart from the World Health Organization (WHO) classification 2020, the ISSVA classification of vascular anomalies encompasses all vascular malformations and tumours in a framework of internationally consistent nomenclature. It divides vascular lesions into vascular tumours and vascular malformations. The vascular tumours may be benign, locally aggressive or borderline and malignant. The vascular surgeons and interventional vascular radiologists use the ISSVA classification extensively whilst diagnosing and treating the vascular lesion. WHO classification is more relevant for diagnosis, treatment and prognosis of the vascular lesions.

TERMINOLOGY

The vascular lesions may demonstrate overlapping imaging features. They are generally classified according to the histological makeup. The "true vascular tumours" demonstrate cellular hyperproliferation and mitosis; e.g. paediatric haemangioma which are subclassified further on the basis of their involution. Conversely, a "vascular malformation" arises from abnormal vascular channels consisting varying degree of arterial, venous and lymphatic components, but endothelial cells turnover is normal.

IMAGING MODALITIES IN VASCULAR LESIONS

Most haemangiomas and vascular malformations are identified according to clinical criteria when superficial. Overlying skin changes and discolouration, location and distribution of the lesion, and age of the patient are important demographic indicators to assess and

DOI: 10.1201/9781003218722-8

differentiate the vascular lesions clinically. However, some deep-seated vascular tumours are challenging to differentiate from other soft tissue sarcomas. The reasons are either an atypical presentation (e.g. soft tissue mass with normal overlying skin) or classification difficulties.

The common lesions include infantile and congenital haemangiomas, which can usually be diagnosed and managed clinically.

● *Plain radiograph*

- Radiographs may be often normal; however, if acoustic shadowing is detected on ultrasound (US) plain radiograph would help in detection of calcification within the soft tissue lesion likely to represent phleboliths. Phleboliths are associated with cavernous haemangiomas in approximately 50% of cases.
- If the mass is large enough and in close proximity to adjacent bone, osseous changes including periosteal reaction and cortical thickening can occur.
- Pressure erosion from the adjacent mass can result in a pathologic fracture.

● *Ultrasound features*

For superficial lesions: High-resolution greyscale and Doppler US allow excellent visualisation of most superficial masses. Doppler US is the easiest way to assess the haemodynamics of a vascular lesion and clarify a doubtful diagnosis between a haemangioma and vascular malformation. US is helpful as it:

- Assesses echogenicity, presence or absence of soft tissue and Doppler flow. Power Doppler study is carried out for detection of disorganised flow.
- Reduces probe pressure on the lesion and reduces Doppler scale to as minimum as possible. US gel-stand-off technique may be helpful to reduce probe pressure optimally for the superficial lesions. Increase colour Doppler gain just up to the start of the speckled artefact and then reduce colour gain which would enable to pick subtle vascularity within the lesion.
- Identifies any evidence of posterior acoustic shadowing to suggest calcification.

Deep-seated lesions: Imaging features are usually indeterminate and appear as ill-defined masses. If the lesion extends below the deep fascia, a cross-sectional imaging, either contrast-enhanced MRI or CT, should be performed.

- The vascular malformations and haemangioma can involve any anatomical location. Vascular malformations should always be in the differentials when one encounters a soft tissue lesion involving multiple compartments, mass effect without significant destruction of underlying muscle, bone or joint.

● *Computed tomography*

Pre- and post-contrast study is done for detection of calcification and assessing enhancement pattern of the lesion. CT is helpful in depicting ill-defined mass of similar attenuation to muscle, intense enhancement following contrast administration and phleboliths which are too small to identify on radiographs.

Serpentine vascular structures may be demonstrated as well as surrounding adipose over-growth. It helps in staging and detection of metastases in aggressive vascular sarcomas.

● *Magnetic resonance imaging*

It is the gold standard for imaging evaluation of soft tissue haemangiomas and vascular tumours. Typically, all sequences show a heterogeneous mass (although lesions measuring less than 2 cm tend to be homogeneous), reflecting the mix of tissues present. MRI supersedes the CT scan due to higher soft tissue resolution, multiplanar acquisition and gadolinium-enhanced images allowing for its extension into the critical structures such as joint and the spinal canal.

T1-weighted images

High-signal-intensity adipose tissue is most prominent along the circumference of the vascular complex. This may reflect muscle atrophy secondary to chronic vascular insufficiency caused by the steal phenomenon. In some patients, the fat overgrowth is so prominent that these lesions are mistaken for lipomas.

T2-weighted images

The central angiomatous core of the neoplasm shows high signal intensity on T2-weighted images. The serpentine nature of the haemangioma, similar to that on contrast-enhanced CT scan, may be depicted on MRI. If blood flow through these vascular channels is rapid enough, the signal may remain low in intensity with all MRI sequences. If gadolinium contrast material is administered, prominent enhancement of the angiomatous tumour is expected.

We will discuss imaging features of a few selected vascular tumours. We have provided exhaustive list of the vascular tumours in Table 8.1 that are categorised according to the latest WHO classification (2020).

Table 8.1: **World Health Organization 2020 Classification of Vascular Tumours**

Benign
Synovial haemangiomas
Intramuscular angioma
Arteriovenous malformation/haemangioma
Venous haemangioma
Anastomosing haemangioma
Epithelioid haemangioma
Lymphangioma and lymphangiomatosis
Intermediate (locally aggressive)
Haemangioendothelioma (Kaposiform, retiform, composite, pseudomyogenic)
Kaposi's sarcoma
Malignant
Angiosarcoma
Dedifferentiated liposarcoma
Perivascular tumours
Glomus tumour
Myopericytoma, angioleioma

BENIGN VASCULAR TUMOURS

● *Haemangioma*

Congenital haemangiomas are most common childhood tumours, occurring in 12% of infants. Haemangiomas are found with greater frequency in girls, whites, premature infants and twins. These lesions can have deep, superficial or mixed components. Most haemangiomas require no therapy. Even many large lesions are treated conservatively because of the characteristic pattern of involution.

Although benign, some haemangiomas may cause life-threatening complications such as Kasabach–Merritt syndrome (consumptive coagulopathy), compression of vital structures (e.g. airway, orbital structures), fissure formation, ulceration and bleeding.

These complications usually occur in the rapid proliferate phase and can be associated with a mortality rate as high as 20 to 30%.

● *Intramuscular angioma/haemangioma*

They are proliferation of benign vascular channels within skeletal muscles, predominantly affecting thigh and calf muscles. The head and neck, upper limb and the trunk are other anatomical sites which are affected in decreasing order. The lesions affect adolescent and young adults preferentially with no gender predisposition. These usually present as slow-growing deep masses which are particularly painful after strenuous activities such as exercise. Larger lesions have potential to induce secondary changes in adjacent bones such osteolysis.

They demonstrate typical imaging features as described below. Superficial lesions also show imaging appearances similar to their intramuscular counterparts.

Imaging features
Ultrasound

Intramuscular haemangioma usually appears as an irregular hyperechoic lesion with variable degree of sinusoidal components without acoustic shadowing. Larger lesions may demonstrate few calcific foci due to phlebolith or metaplastic ossification. It may demonstrate punctate foci of internal flow on colour Doppler imaging.

● *MRI*

It demonstrates intermediate signal between that of muscle and fat and, in some cases, peripheral high-signal-intensity areas representing intralesional fat on T1-weighted imaging (Figure 8.1). Larger lesions may demonstrate adjacent muscle atrophy due to long-standing mass effect on muscle fascicles and fatty proliferation.

On T2-weighted images, it appears as a well-defined slightly hyperintense lesion containing multiple high-signal-intensity lobules resembling a bunch of grapes. This appearance is due to cavernous or cystic vascular spaces containing stagnant blood (Figure 8.2). Punctate or reticular low-signal-intensity areas may be present, representing fibrous tissue, fast flow within vessels or foci of calcification. Areas of thrombosis appear as circular low-signal-intensity areas on all MR sequences similar to phleboliths which would be difficult to differentiate on MRI alone. Plain radiographs would be helpful in such circumstances.

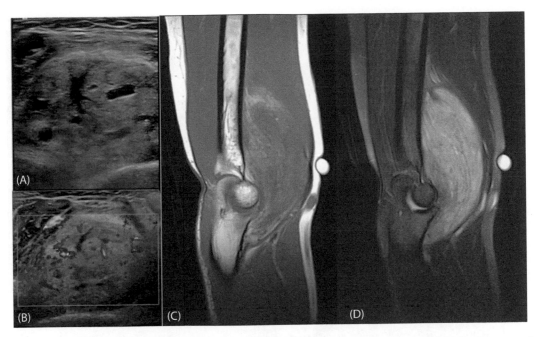

Figure 8.1: Intramuscular haemangioma. Greyscale (A) and colour Doppler (B) ultrasound images show a deep solid mixed echogenicity mass lesion within the brachialis muscle with marked echogenicity and traversing vascular channels. T1-weighted (C) and STIR (D) images depict diffuse hypertrophy of the involved brachialis muscle which shows increased STIR signal. The most important feature is preservation of the fat between the muscle fibres with tiny vessels criss-crossing the lesion. Intramuscular haemangiomas are often associated with genetic mutations which lead to localised hypertrophy of the involved muscle and fatty tissue. (Image Courtesy of Dr. Harun Gupta.)

Post-contrast maximum intensity projection images can identify feeding vessels which may help in further management (Figure 8.3).

● *Synovial haemangioma*

It is a rare subset of haemangioma which almost always involves the knee joint. The patient usually presents with pain, swelling and joint effusion. The most common site of involvement is the suprapatellar pouch (Figure 8.4). Imaging features are similar to that of a soft tissue haemangioma but may be mistaken for other nodular lesions in view of its location. It can demonstrate extra-articular involvement and cause pressure erosions of adjacent bone.

● *Lymphangioma*

A lymphangioma in adults, also known as a cystic hygroma in infants, is a benign localised collection of the dilated lymphatic channels. It can be solitary or multicentric, superficial or deep and can involve the head and neck, extremities, axilla and groin. If multicentric and involving multiple organs traversing through different tissue planes, it is known as lymphangiomatosis. It presents as soft, painless and fluctuant swelling. Superimposed infection or internal bleeding can occur especially following trauma.

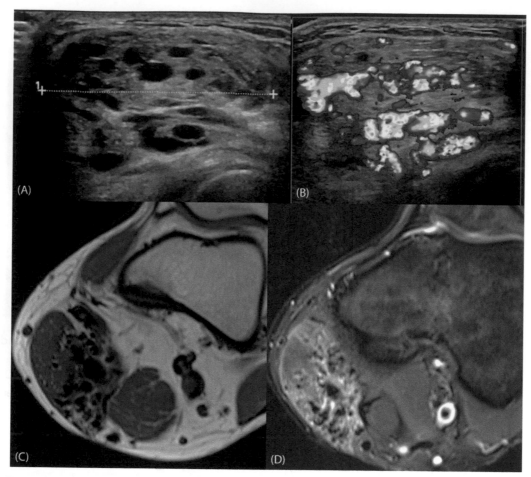

Figure 8.2: Arteriovenous haemangioma. Greyscale (A) and colour Doppler (B) ultrasound images demonstrate complex solid-cystic mass lesion with echogenic solid component infiltrated extensively by vascular channels. These vascular feeds show high blood flow on Doppler imaging. T1-weighted (C) and STIR (D) images show sizable solid component. Such tumours require collaborative approach involving both sarcoma team and interventional vascular radiologists for further management.

Imaging features of lymphangioma are non-specific. On US, it appears as a lobulated, anechoic mass (Figure 8.5A and B) which may contain internal septae and septal vascularity. Internal debris (chylous component) and soft tissue component may occur. On CT, it usually shows cystic density but variation in density may occur based upon its blood, fat and proteinaceous contents. It appears bright on T2-weighted and STIR images and shows variable signal intensity on T1-weighted images depending upon its fluid content. On post-gadolinium images, it shows thin peripheral enhancement. Septae may also enhance (Figure 8.5C–E).

INTERMEDIATE VASCULAR TUMOURS

● *Haemangioendothelioma*

There are numerous subtypes of haemangioendotheliomas depending upon their histological makeup. Tufted/Kaposiform haemangioendothelioma are most common. It is a rare

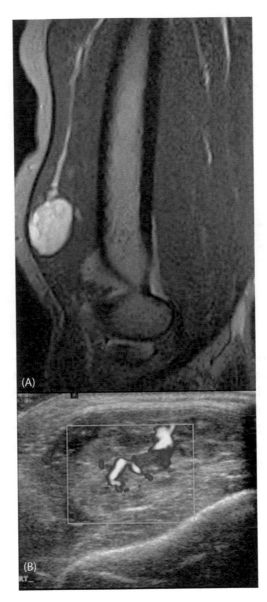

Figure 8.3: Feeding vessel in a haemangioma. Contrast-enhanced T1-weighted image (A) depict a blood vessel feeding the intensely enhancing intramuscular angioma/haemangioma in the arm. Corresponding Doppler ultrasound image (B) shows marked internal vascularity. (Image Courtesy of: Dr Harun Gupta, Consultant MSK radiologist, Leeds, UK)

disease of childhood. There is no gender predilection and most commonly presents in the first year of life, but there are reports of development in later life also.

Imaging features are non-specific (Figure 8.6). The lesions mimic haemangiomas. If larger, it appears as an ill-defined hyperechoic mass with increased vascularity on US. On CT, it demonstrates a homogenous mass with ill-defined margins showing iso-attenuation to adjacent muscles on unenhanced CT and heterogenous enhancement on post-contrast images. It often shows extension into surrounding structures. It appears hypointense on T1-weighted images and heterogeneously hyperintense on T2-weighted and post-contrast images.

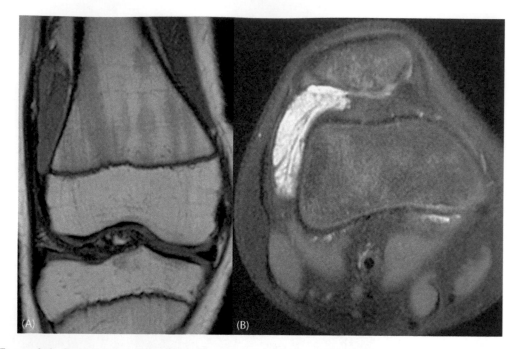

Figure 8.4: Synovial haemangioma. Large intra-articular soft tissue mass lesion demonstrates indeterminate yet non-aggressive features. T1-weighted coronal (A) and STIR axial (B) images show a solid lesion (hyperintense on T1-weighted and STIR) within the lateral recess of the suprapatellar pouch with well-demarked margins, no soft tissue or bone infiltration or other aggressive features like haemorrhage, necrotic or cystic components. The knee is the most common anatomical site for the synovial haemangioma. (Image Courtesy of Dr. Harun Gupta.)

Kaposi's sarcoma

Kaposi's sarcoma (KS) represents a virus-induced locally aggressive vascular proliferation. It is universally associated with HHV-8 virus. Skin is the most common site affected; however, mucous membranes, lymph nodes and visceral organs can also be affected. There are four distinct subtypes: classic KS, endemic KS, transplant-associated KS and HIV-related KS. HIV-associated KS is the most aggressive form when untreated.

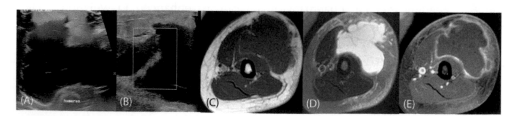

Figure 8.5: Lymphangioma. Greyscale (A) and colour Doppler (B) images demonstrate a large lobulated marginated cystic lesion involving the arm with absent internal vascularity. The patient has complained about increase in size following recent trauma in a long-standing swelling for more than 20 years (since childhood). T1-weighted (C), STIR (D) and post-contrast fat-suppressed T1-weighted (E) images showing characteristic cystic lesion (hypointense on T1-weighted and hyperintense on STIR) with very fine septae but absent solid component. It shows peripheral thin-rim enhancement. (Image Courtesy of Dr. Harun Gupta.)

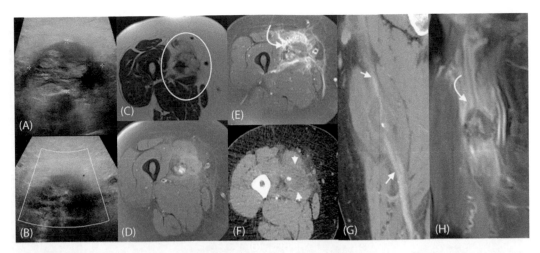

Figure 8.6: Haemangioendothelioma. Greyscale (A) and colour Doppler (B) ultrasound images showing a large aggressive appearing deep solid mass lesion in the right midthigh in a patient with previous history of breast carcinoma. The lesion has raised a suspicion of metastatic deposit. Corresponding T1-weighted (C) and STIR (D) images show an ill-marginated locally aggressive soft tissue mass lesion (white circle) with foci of calcification encasing the superficial femoral artery and vein with adjacent muscle oedema (curved arrows). The lesion showed a large non-enhancing component (arrowheads) around the involved vessel on both contrast-enhanced axial MRI (E), axial (F) and MIP CT (G) and coronal MRI (H). Sagittal MIP reformatted contrast-enhanced CT image showed the lesion circumferentially involving the superficial femoral artery (arrows) with luminal narrowing and foci of calcification. It was subsequently biopsied (not shown) and proven to be haemangioendothelioma. (Image Courtesy of Dr Katalin Boros and Dr Siddharth Thaker.)

Imaging is predominantly helpful in diagnosing visceral KS affecting the lungs and abdominal organs. KS affecting skin is a dermatological diagnosis. US can show skin thickening with increased blood flow on Doppler imaging. MRI may be helpful in detecting deep-seated lesions affecting musculoskeletal system. MRI features are non-specific (Figure 8.7) and biopsy is generally required for the final diagnosis.

MALIGNANT VASCULAR TUMOURS

Angiosarcoma

It is a rare and highly aggressive tumour that can affect any organ in the body. It most commonly presents in its cutaneous form (nearly 50%). It predominantly affects older males in their 60 to 70s. It has a poor prognosis, particularly when the patient is diagnosed with metastases at initial presentation, as is often the case. The head and neck are the most common anatomical site affected. In the early stages, it can be misdiagnosed for benign entities caused by cellulitis, infection or skin injuries. As the tumour size increases, ulceration, haemorrhage and oedema can develop. Even with radical surgical resection, positive margins and local recurrence is common.

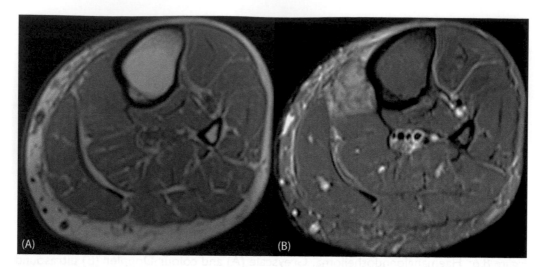

Figure 8.7: Kaposi's sarcoma. T1-weighted (A) and STIR (B) images demonstrate a deep intramuscular solid lesion within the soleus muscle medially. The lesion shows isointense signal on T1-weighted image and increased STIR signal. Kaposi's sarcoma can virtually involve any tissue but has an affinity for the skin. Kaposi's sarcoma should always be included in the differential when presented with an atypical soft tissue mass in an immunocompromised patient. (Image Courtesy of Dr. Harun Gupta.)

On US, appearances are usually indeterminate and may show areas of diffuse subcutaneous oedema with increased vascularity which may be mistaken as underlying acute inflammatory or infective changes. Contrast-enhanced CT scan may demonstrate irregular, enhancing soft tissue mass in early cases and underlying bone or adjacent solid organ invasion in advanced cases. Soft tissue calcifications can also be seen.

MRI (Figure 8.8) is helpful in defining the size and extent of the lesion and involvement of the anatomical structures. Angiosarcoma appears with intermediate signal intensity on T1-weighted images often intermixed with foci of high signal intensity from haemorrhage. On T2-weighted image, it appears bright with vessels within the tumour showing either high flow (low signal intensity on all pulse sequences) or low flow (increased signal intensity on T2-weighted images). It appears heterogenous following gadolinium due to internal necrotic areas.

The most diagnostic finding is the presence of high-flow serpentine vessels in an otherwise solid non-specific heterogenous soft tissue mass.

Angiosarcoma shows avid fluorine-18 fludeoxyglucose (18F-FDG) uptake on positron emission tomography (PET)-CT. PET-CT can differentiate radiation-induced skin necrosis from recurrence (Figure 8.9).

Metastatic potential: It has a high tendency to be haematogenous metastatic multifocal and therefore aggressive disease. The lungs are most commonly involved. Other sites include the liver, bone and lymph nodes. Angiosarcoma should be considered in the differential diagnosis if imaging shows metastatic disease in the lungs with nodules and cysts surrounded with ground-glass opacification and hydropneumothorax.

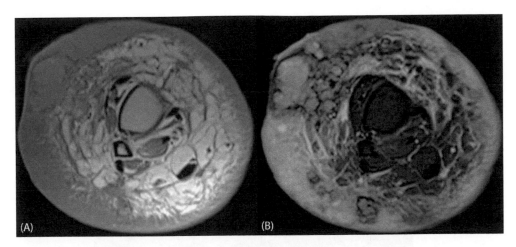

Figure 8.8: Angiosarcoma. T1-weighted (A) and STIR (B) axial images at the level of the left tibial midshaft show a diffuse abnormality centred over the subdermal region of the entire subcutaneous layer. It forms a heterogenous soft tissue mass anteriorly with background of extensive soft tissue oedema. The mass-like soft tissue component was target for ultrasound-guided biopsy which turned out to be an angiosarcoma. (Image Courtesy of Dr. Harun Gupta.)

VASCULAR TUMOUR-LIKE CONDITIONS

● *Arteriovenous malformations (Figure 8.10)*

Slow-flow vascular malformations (venous, capillary, cavernous or mixed) contain large spaces with fine serpentine structures that are usually oriented along the long axis of the extremities; these follow a neurovascular bundle and are sometimes multifocal. They are classified on the basis of predominant vessel type. High-flow vascular malformations show more prominent serpentine vessels. Faster flow may manifest as areas of flow void with all pulse sequences. Digital subtraction angiography serves as a modality of choice for diagnostic and management purpose.

PERIVASCULAR LESIONS MIMICKING VASCULAR TUMOURS (GLOMUS TUMOUR)

Glomus tumour, otherwise known as a glomangioma, is a benign perivascular tissue proliferation predominantly affecting young-to-middle aged individuals (fourth–sixth decade of life). There is slight female preponderance. More than 75% lesions occur in hands and subungal location is considered characteristic. It presents as a painful, reddish-blue mass beneath the nail bed or around the tuft of the digit which is remarkably symptomatic during the night.

On US it appears as a hypoechoic nodular mass lesion showing intense vascularity and, often, pressure effect leading cortical erosion of the adjacent bone (Figure 8.11). It generally

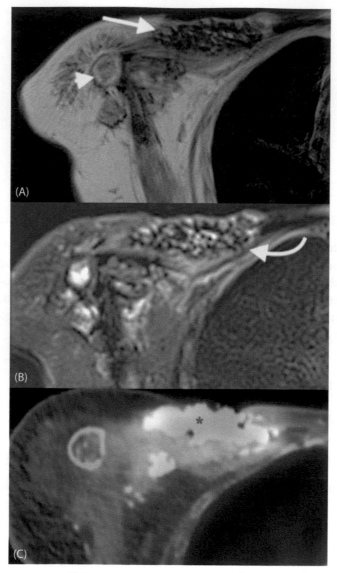

Figure 8.9: Radiobionecrosis in a treated angiosarcoma. The patient has history of angiosarcoma which was excised with narrow margins and subsequently treated with adjuvant radiotherapy. T1-weighted (A) and STIR (B) axial images at the level of right anterior chest wall and axilla demonstrate diffuse soft tissue oedema (curved arrow) surrounding sizable area of diffuse T1-weighted and STIR hypointense signal. Such MRI appearances pose diagnostic dilemma between post-radiotherapy changes versus recurrence. Also appreciate increased STIR signal with corresponding low signal on T1-weighted image from extensive osteonecrosis of the humeral head up to surgical neck (arrowhead) and acute on chronic (mixed oedema and fatty atrophy) shoulder girdle muscle changes due to their involvement in the radiation field. PET-CT (C) demonstrated extensive calcification (asterisk) corresponding to diffuse low MRI signal and lack of intense radiotracer uptake favouring post-treatment changes. Ultrasound-guided biopsy from the margin of the treated area showed inflammatory changes, intermixed fibrotic tissue and absence of sarcomatous tissue. (Image Courtesy of Dr Harun Gupta and Dr Siddharth Thaker.)

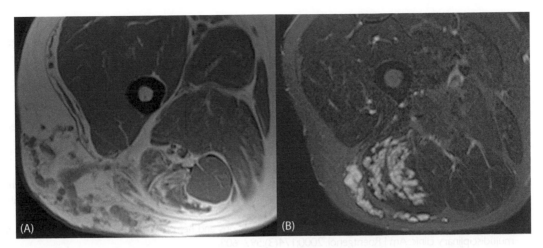

Figure 8.10: Vascular malformation. T1-weighted (A) and STIR (B) axial MRI images at the mid-thigh level demonstrate convoluted vascular channels predominantly affecting the posterior muscle compartment of the thigh. There is predominant involvement of the biceps femoris muscle without apparent soft tissue mass. Vascular malformations, contrary to true vascular tumours, typically lack the endothelial overgrowth. Hence, their treatment differs from true vascular tumours. (Image Courtesy of Dr. Harun Gupta.)

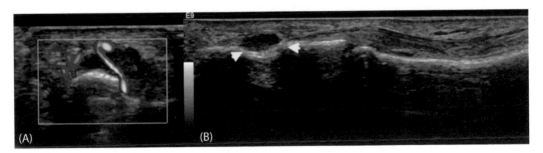

Figure 8.11: Glomus tumour. Short-axis colour Doppler (A) and long-axis greyscale panoramic ultrasound (B) images show a small hypervascular mass indenting the cortex of the distal phalanx – a characteristic location for the glomus tumour. (Image Courtesy of Dr. Harun Gupta.)

shows iso- to hypointensity on T1-weighted images, marked hyperintensity on T2-weighted images and intense enhancement following gadolinium administration.

Take-home points

- Doppler US and MRI are the two main imaging modalities that allow classification of the vascular anomalies and are useful in those clinically uncertain cases to establish the correct diagnosis.
- Presence of fat, calcification and signal voids in the lesion help in steering the diagnosis towards a vascular lesion.
- Necrosis and more diffuse pattern of involvement favour aggressive lesion.
- PET-CT imaging are useful in characterising lesions when in doubt, staging and post-treatment work up of aggressive vascular lesions.

- Metastasis is usually the initial presentation in angiosarcomas. Although prognosis is poor, the radiologist can aid in diagnosis, staging and image-guided interventions after discussion with the multidisciplinary team.

SUGGESTED READING

- Bansal, A, Goyal, S, Goyal, A, Jana, M. WHO classification of soft tissue tumours 2020: An update and simplified approach for radiologists. Eur J Radiol. 2021;143:109937.
- Bhaludin, BN, Thway, K, Adejolu, M, Renn, A, Kelly-Morland, C, Fisher, C, Jones, RL, Messiou, C, Moskovic, E. Imaging features of primary sites and metastatic patterns of angiosarcoma. Insights Imag. 2021;12(1):1–8.
- Croteau, SE, Liang, MG, Kozakewich, HP, Alomari, AI, Fishman, SJ, Mulliken, JB, Trenor, CC III. Kaposiform hemangioendothelioma: Atypical features and risks of Kasabach-Merritt phenomenon in 107 referrals. J Pediatr. 2013;162(1):142–147.
- Donnelly, LF, Adams, DM, Bisset, GS III. Vascular malformations and hemangiomas: A practical approach in a multidisciplinary clinic. Am J Roentgenol. 2000;174(3):597–608.
- Flors, L, Leiva-Salinas, C, Norton, PT, Park, AW, Ogur, T, Hagspiel, KD. Ten frequently asked questions about MRI evaluation of soft-tissue vascular anomalies. Am J Roentgenol. 2013;201(4):W554–562.
- Jang, JK, Thomas, R, Braschi-Amirfarzan, M, Jagannathan, JP. A review of the spectrum of imaging manifestations of epithelioid hemangioendothelioma. Am J Roentgenol. 2020;215(5):1290–1298.
- Khosa, F, Magoon, P, Bedi, H, Khan, AN, Otero, H, Yucel, K. Primary and metastatic vascular neoplasms: Imaging findings. Am J Roentgenol. 2012;198(3):700–704.
- Olsen, KI, Stacy, GS, Montag, A. Soft-tissue cavernous hemangioma. Radiographics. 2004;24(3):849–854.

9 Tumours of uncertain origin

Aanand Vibhakar,
Winston Rennie, Amit Shah

INTRODUCTION

Certain soft tissue tumours have phenotypes that do not conform to a defined tissue type or lack clear differentiation towards a defined mesenchymal tissue type. These tumours are currently regarded as tumours of uncertain differentiation.

Despite being challenging to diagnose, there have been advances in the understanding of their genetic and pathologic features. Understanding the molecular genetics of tumours improves the diagnostic accuracy for tumours with overlapping morphological features or that have been difficult to classify on the basis of morphology alone.

The latest World Health Organization (WHO) 2020 classification for soft tissue and bone tumours divides tumours of uncertain differentiation into an extensive list divided into four categories (Table 9.1) based on their molecular genetics, immunohistochemistry and histopathological features.

Although many of these tumours may be challenging to identify based on imaging alone, the radiologist must be aware of the updated changes.

A major update is the removal of undifferentiated/unclassified tumours as a separate category and their merger into tumours of uncertain differentiation. In addition, acral fibromyxoma has been removed from tumours of uncertain differentiation and reclassified as a benign fibroblastic tumour.

This chapter provides an overview on the radiological manifestations of tumours of uncertain differentiation, highlights key changes in the new 2020 WHO classification and focuses on selected tumours.

IMAGING MODALITIES IN TUMOURS OF UNCERTAIN DIFFERENTIATION

● Ultrasound

- Ultrasound has a limited role as most of these tumours arise in deep soft tissues for which MRI is a superior imaging modality. For superficial lesions arising in the extremities, ultrasound can assess whether a lesion appears aggressive or non-aggressive.

DOI: 10.1201/9781003218722-9

Table 9.1: **Tumours of Uncertain Differentiation (WHO 2020 Classification)**

Benign
Myxoma
Aggressive angiomyxoma
Pleomorphic hyalinizing angiectatic tumour
Phosphaturic mesenchymal tumour
Perivascular epithelioid tumour
Angiomyolipoma
Locally aggressive
Epithelioid angiomyolipoma
Haemosiderotic fibrolipomatous tumour
Rarely metastasising
Atypical fibroxanthoma
Angiomatoid fibrous histiocytoma
Ossifying fibromyxoid tumour
Myoepithelioma
Malignant
NTRK Rearranged spindle cell neoplasm
Synovial Sarcoma
Epithelioid sarcoma
Alveolar soft part sarcoma
Clear cell sarcoma
Extra-skeletal myxoid chondrosarcoma
Desmoplastic small round cell tumour
Rhabdoid tumour
Malignant perivascular epithelioid tumour
Intimal sarcoma
Malignant ossifying fibromyxoid tumour
Undifferentiated sarcoma
Undifferentiated spindle cell sarcoma
Undifferentiated pleomorphic sarcoma

- Ultrasound can assess the nature (i.e. solid versus cystic), size, shape, margins, number, vascularity, location (superficial vs. deep to deep fascia) and anatomical relationships to adjoining structures.
- Ultrasound is the modality of choice for image-guided biopsy of soft tissue lesions.

● *Magnetic resonance imaging*

- Magnetic resonance imaging (MRI) is the imaging modality of choice for characterising tumours of uncertain differentiation and delineating anatomical boundaries of complex lesions.
- MRI is required for pre-surgical evaluation, particularly to identify the relationship with neurovascular structures, anatomical compartments, fascial or osseous involvement.
- MRI is vital for post-surgical monitoring and evaluating local complications and recurrence.

- Whole-body MRI is becoming more popular for staging tumours rather than computed tomography (CT), though its use is variable due to economic, logistical and specialist factors.

Computed tomography

- CT is predominantly used when MRI is contraindicated or for disease staging.
- CT is useful for the assessment of calcification or ossification of a lesion.
- Extra-skeletal myxoid chondrosarcoma can exhibit periosteal reaction, bone erosion and invasion.
- Malignant ossifying fibromyxoid tumour has variable central and peripheral mineralisation when differentials of myositis ossificans or synovial sarcoma are considered.
- Staging CT chest is essential in the work-up of clear cell sarcoma and synovial sarcoma, where lung metastases are common.
- CT can also be used for image-guided biopsy, particularly of deeper lesions that cannot be safely targeted with ultrasound (i.e. the intercondylar notch).

Positron emission tomography-CT

- There is no currently established role for PET-CT in imaging these tumours in particular.
- Case reports have described the use of PET-CT in assessing disease extent before consideration of tumour resection and in its use for assessment of disease recurrence.

For ease of understanding and congruence, we will discuss the radiological appearances of tumours of uncertain differentiation according to their categorisation in the latest WHO 2020 classification.

BENIGN TUMOURS OF UNCERTAIN DIFFERENTIATION

Angiomyolipoma

Angiomyolipoma is a new introduction into this category in the latest WHO 2020 guidelines. Most of these occur sporadically; a small subset is associated with tuberous sclerosis. It can occur anywhere in the body but is most commonly seen in the extremities, particularly the lower leg, and it shows vascular, fatty and muscle components. Due to very few reported cases and non-specific imaging findings, there are no specifically recognised imaging features.

Myxoma

Most myxomas occur in intramuscular sites (Figure 9.1A), although they may also be subcutaneous, intermuscular or juxta-articular. Myxomas typically present as slow-growing, painless masses. They can occur sporadically or in Mazabraud syndrome together with fibrous dysplasia (Figure 9.1B). They are usually diagnosed in middle age and are more common in women. Classic intramuscular myxoma is typically a non-recurrent tumour, whereas the cellular subtype has a small risk for local recurrence.

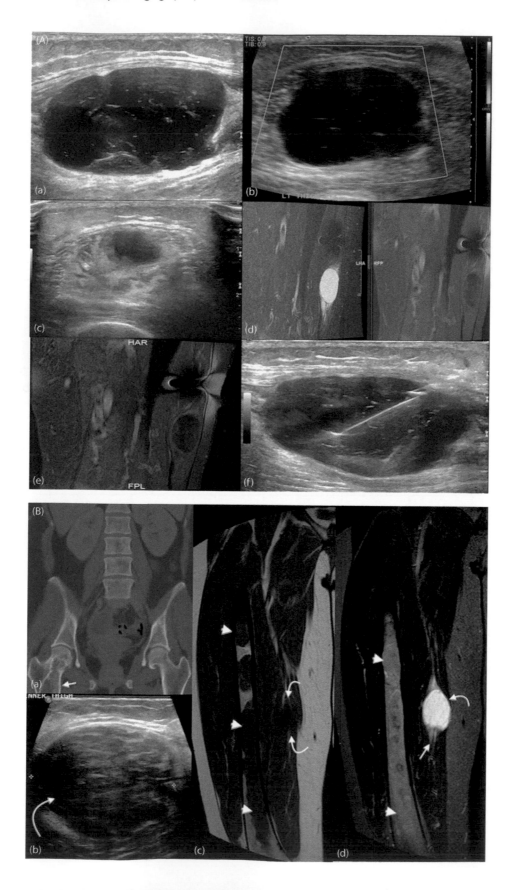

Ultrasound features

They usually present as well-circumscribed masses, and their echogenicity varies from heterogeneously hypoechoic to near anechoic and demonstrate increased through transmission and small anechoic cystic areas with bright rim of increased echogenicity around the lesion corresponding to fat.

CT features

The attenuation varies between fluid and muscle. They demonstrate mild diffuse enhancement or peripheral and septal enhancement in 50% cases.

MRI features

They are homogenous to mildly heterogeneous and may contain septae or cystic foci. On T1-weighted (T1W) images, they demonstrate low (81–100%) to intermediate (0–19%) signal intensity. They have a characteristic rim of fat usually seen around the lesion's superior and inferior poles, which may represent fatty atrophy of adjacent muscle. On fluid-sensitive sequences, they demonstrate high signal intensity. High signal in the surrounding tissues from leakage of myxomatous tissue is common, with flame or brush-like appearances along longitudinal muscle fascicles. Cystic foci are seen in 50% of cases. They demonstrate mild to moderate enhancement. They either demonstrate diffuse or thick and peripheral septal enhancement. Regions of globular enhancement have also been described.

● *Aggressive angiomyxoma*

It is an infiltrative, benign, myxoid spindle cell neoplasm that occurs in the deep soft tissue of the pelviperineal region, including the vulvovaginal and inguinoscrotal soft tissue in women and men, respectively. They present as slow-growing, deep-seated painless masses. Clinically they can be confused with pelvic abscesses, Bartholin gland cysts, hernias or adnexal masses. They have a wide age range, with a peak in the fourth to fifth decade and are much more common in women. Recurrence rates vary, ranging from 9 to 50%.

Figure 9.1: (A) Intramuscular myxoma. Longitudinal ultrasound through the left upper thigh (a) reveals a hypoechoic lesion with a few low-level internal echoes. Doppler ultrasound of the same lesion (b) shows no vascularity. A longitudinal ultrasound view with an increased time gain compensation (c) reveals a part-solid solid nature of the previously thought "cystic" lesion. Coronal STIR (left) and T1 fat-saturated contrast-enhanced images (right) (d) demonstrate an intramuscular cystic lesion with faint peripheral enhancement. This is further demonstrated on post-contrast images (e). An aggressive process could not be excluded on ultrasound or MRI, and an ultrasound-guided biopsy (f) was performed. Histopathology supported a diagnosis of a benign intramuscular myxoma. (B) Mazabraud syndrome. Coronal CT image (a) shows well-marginated bony lesion with ground-glass matrix (straight arrow) causing mild bony expansion consistent with fibrous dysplasia. Please appreciate similar changes in the lumbar vertebrae. The patient complaints of a soft tissue mass lesion in the right medial thigh which on greyscale ultrasound (b) image shows an intramuscular mass lesion (curved arrow). Subsequent coronal T1-weighted (c) and STIR (d) images confirm multiple bony lesions consistent with fibrous dysplasia (arrowheads) involving the right femur and an intramuscular myxoma (curved arrows) and a characteristic myxoid tail (straight arrow) at the margins. (Image Courtesy of Dr. Harun Gupta.)

Ultrasound features

The mass may appear hypoechoic or cystic.

CT features

Lesions demonstrate a variable morphology ranging from a hypo- or isodense mass demonstrating post-contrast enhancement. A swirled appearance can often be seen.

MRI features

Lesions are usually T1 isointense to muscle and T2 hyperintense with internal areas of whorled linear T1 and T2 hypointense signal. The swirled appearance is most likely due to the fibrovascular stroma which gets stretched as the mass extends to involve the pelvic diaphragm. Post-contrast T1W image also demonstrates the swirled appearance. Infiltration into the pelvic floor muscles or perineum is best evaluated using MRI.

● *Phosphaturic mesenchymal tumour*

Phosphaturic mesenchymal tumours (PMTs, Figure 9.2) have been reclassified from the rarely metastasising category into benign and malignant subtypes based on histological features. They are morphologically distinctive neoplasms that frequently cause tumour-induced osteomalacia (TIO), a rare paraneoplastic syndrome. Metabolic disturbances can lead to hypophosphatemia, osteomalacia, rickets and secondary hyperparathyroidism. Adult patients may complain of chronic hypophosphatemia symptoms, including bone and muscle pain, malaise and muscle stiffness. PMTs commonly affect middle-aged adults of either sex (M:F = 1:1) but these can also occur in paediatric or elderly patients. Their aetiology is unknown.

The vast majority of PMTs are histologically benign. Complete excision can result in dramatic improvement of phosphate wasting and osteomalacia. However, malignant tumours may metastasise and cause death.

Chart 9.1 describes a suggested imaging pathway for the investigation of PMTs.

Radiographic features

Radiographic findings include cortical thinning, coarse trabeculations and Looser's zones in adults, and features of rickets in children. Non-united osteopenic fractures are also commonly demonstrated in the foot and pelvis.

CT features

On CT, PMTs may demonstrate an internal matrix with a punctated or amorphous appearance. Less commonly, they may exhibit a ground-glass matrix. PMTs affecting the bone are commonly lytic; however, sclerotic and mixed lytic and sclerotic appearances have also been observed.

MRI features

Variable appearances have been reported on MRI. Generally, PMTs exhibit an iso- to hyperintense signal on T1W images and a hyperintense signal on T2W images. T2 hyperintense signal with internal hypointense foci or vascular flow voids can be observed in larger masses. Commonly PMTs demonstrate homogenous or peripheral contrast enhancement in smaller lesions and heterogeneous enhancement in larger lesions. Internal haemorrhage, fluid-fluid levels and surrounding oedematous change have also been described.

Radionuclide imaging features

Radionuclide imaging has shown increasing promise in localising lesions in cases of TIO. Seventy-nine per cent of surface receptors on PMTs have been shown to express

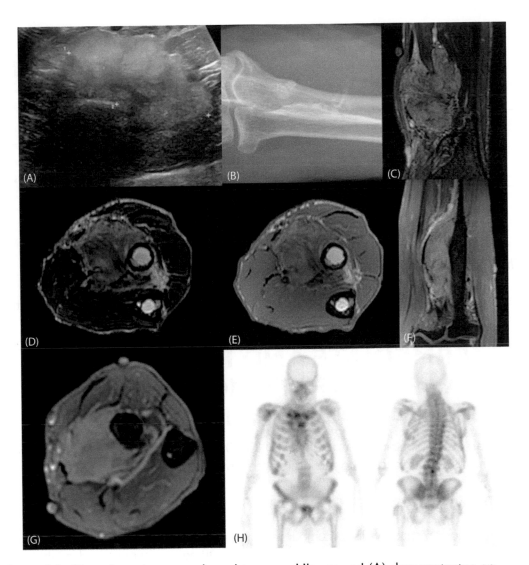

Figure 9.2: Phosphaturic mesenchymal tumour. Ultrasound (A) demonstrates an irregular, heterogenous lesion with internal predominantly hyperechoic components in the flexor compartment of the right proximal forearm. Calcification within the lesion is seen on radiographs (B). Sagittal TI (C), axial T2 (D), axial TI (E), coronal TI post-contrast (F) and axial TI post-contrast (G) MRI images reveals a solid, aggressive enhancing intermuscular lesion intimately wrapped around the periosteum of the proximal radius. Tc99 MDP bone scan (H) reveals multiple bilateral foci of increased tracer uptake in the ribs in keeping with old rib fractures. Focal osteopenia at both proximal femora are from bilateral total hip replacements secondary to fractures. Multiple skeletal fractures are a manifestation of tumour induced osteomalacia, a common manifestation of phosphaturic mesenchymal tumour.

somatostatin. Thus, somatostatin analogues can be used to search for PMT in cases of TIO. 18F-FDG PET can also be useful with most PMTs demonstrating moderate FDG avidity with an average SUVmax of 4.1. Case reports suggest that 99Tc-HYNIC-TOC SPECT/CT and 68 Ga-DOTATATE PET/CT are the most effective radionuclide investigations for identifying a PMT. Functional whole-body imaging is recommended to effectively localise lesions before

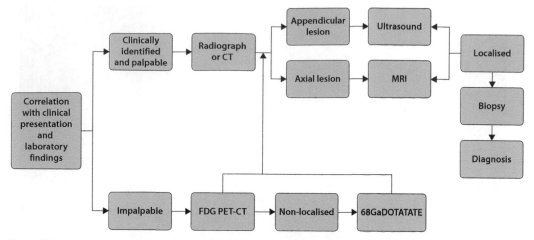

Chart 9.1: Imaging pathway for phosphaturic mesenchymal tumours.

definitive treatment due to their variable size and location. Management is surgical resection with serial post-operative blood tests, including serum phosphate and FGF-23 levels.

INTERMEDIATE AND RARELY METASTASISING TUMOURS OF UNCERTAIN DIFFERENTIATION

These are listed in Table 9.1. In the new WHO 2020 classification, epithelioid angiomyolipoma has been introduced into the locally aggressive category.

● *Malignant tumours of uncertain differentiation*

These include an extensive list of tumours as listed in Table 9.1. A few selected tumours will be discussed here, and an overview of the rest of the tumours is summarised in Table 9.2.

NTRK-rearranged spindle cell neoplasm

NTRK-rearranged spindle cell neoplasm is an emerging entity and a new addition to the malignant category in the new WHO 2020 classification. It occurs in young adults.

NTRK-rearranged spindle cell neoplasms (outside infantile fibrosarcomas) constitute an emerging group of molecularly defined rare soft tissue tumours. Most present as superficial or deep tumours in the extremities or trunk as a palpable, non-tender mass. Most occur in the first two decades of life, with lipofibromatosis-like neural tumours presenting predominantly in children with a median age of 13.5 years. Tumours with high-grade morphological features may show aggressive clinical behaviour with metastatic spread to the lungs and other organs.

There are no established imaging findings for these lesions.

Synovial sarcoma

Synovial sarcomas (SS, Figure 9.3A) are monomorphic blue spindle cell sarcomas. The majority (70%) arise in the deep soft tissue of the lower and upper extremities. Fifteen per cent arise in the trunk and 7% in the head and neck. They usually present as a swelling which may be painful. They may occur at any age and have no gender predilection. Over half of patients

Table 9.2: An Overview of the Rest of the Malignant Tumours of Uncertain Differentiation

Tumour	Clinical features	Imaging findings
Epithelioid sarcoma	It is the most common hand and wrist malignancy in patients of 6–25 years of age. Patients can present with solitary or multiple firm, painless nodules and non-healing skin ulcers. The conventional (distal) type occurs in patients of 10–35 years of age and the proximal type occur in older adults. The proximal type tumours are located in the deep soft tissue. Usually larger in size and more infiltrative.	**Anatomical sites: Conventional (distal) type:** 60% involve the flexor surface of the distal upper extremity. It has a tendency to propagate along fascia, tendon sheaths, nerve sheaths and metastasise to the lymphatics. **Proximal type:** the pelvis, perineum and genital tract are affected in decreasing order of frequency. **MRI:** homogenously isointense to muscle on T1, heterogeneously hyperintense on fluid-sensitive sequences, and commonly exhibits internal necrosis and peripheral high signal oedema. Enhances heterogeneously.
Clear cell sarcoma	Malignant mesenchymal tumour with melanocytic differentiation and a nested growth pattern, typically occurring in deep soft tissues. Occur in young adults, with a slight female predominance. Peak incidence in the 3rd and 4th decades of life. Aggressive malignancy with recurrence rates of nearly 40% and pulmonary or lymph node metastases. Metastasis often occur more than a decade after initial diagnosis. Tumour size >5 cm, necrosis and regional lymph node involvement are poor prognostic features.	**Anatomical sites:** typically involve tendons and aponeuroses of extremities, particularly the ankle and foot. **MRI:** slightly hyperintense to muscle on T1W images likely due to the presence of melanin and markedly hyperintense to muscle on T2W images. It has been suggested that clear cell sarcoma should be suspected in a lesion that displays high signal intensity on all sequences including fat-saturated sequences. They can be difficult to differentiate from malignant melanoma.
Extrarenal rhabdoid tumour	Extremely rare. Occurs in infants and young children. Most commonly present as a rapidly enlarging soft tissue mass.	**Anatomical sites:** paraspinal region, neck, perineum, pelvic cavity, retroperitoneum and abdominal cavity. **Radiographs:** aggressive lobulated, soft tissue masses with bone erosion. **MRI:** lobulated, irregular and heterogeneous masses on T1W, T2W and contrast-enhanced images.
Malignant perivascular epithelioid cell tumour (PEComas)	They are rare tumours, and more frequent in females with a broad age-peak in young to middle-aged adults. Most PEComas are sporadic; a small subset is associated with tuberous sclerosis	Due to very few reported cases, no specific imaging features are recognised
Malignant ossifying fibromyxoid tumour	Rare tumour. Painless, slow-growing mass in the extremity. Median age of presentation 50 years (range 14–79). Male predominance	**Ultrasound:** lesions are well-circumscribed, hypoechoic and avascular. **Radiographs and CT:** a soft tissue mass with periosteal reaction, central and peripheral calcification or ossification. **MRI:** heterogeneous signal on T1W, fluid-sensitive and enhanced sequences. Foci of high T1 signal fatty marrow in regions of ossification. **NM Scan:** intense Tc-99m MDP and avid F-18 FDG uptake

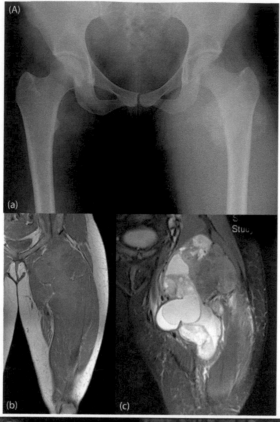

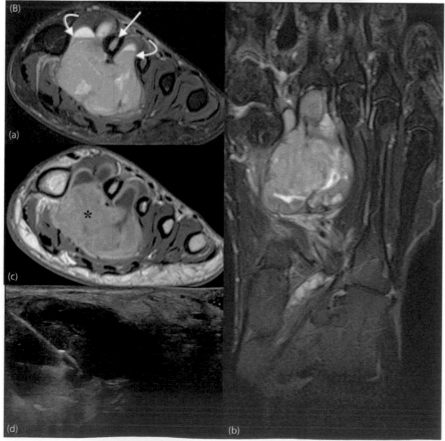

are adolescents or young adults. SS is associated with a history of the previous radiotherapy. Most are 3 to 10 cm in diameter at diagnosis. Small lesions (<1 cm) tend to occur in the hands and feet. SS is frequently multinodular, can be multicystic, shows calcification, metaplastic ossification and necrosis, and has a variable prognosis. The metastatic disease often affects the lungs, bones and regional lymph nodes. Children fare better than adults and extremity-based SSs have a better prognosis than SSs involving the head and neck or trunk.

CT features
Heterogenous mass often occurs in a juxta-articular location (usually the popliteal fossa of the knee) or tendon sheath but almost never in intra-articular location. Up to 95% occur in the extremities (lower > upper). They may have stippled or spiculated forms of calcification (calcification seen in a third of cases). SS with aggressive growth may erode or invade adjacent bone (11–25%). Attenuation on CT is similar to or lower than muscle.

MRI features
Heterogenous MRI signals from haemosiderin, cystic change and fluid-fluid levels are common (Figure 9.3B). Lesions demonstrate prominent heterogeneous enhancement. Classically on T2W images, SS demonstrates the triple sign (multiple signal intensities from haemorrhage, solid tissue, necrosis and calcification) and the bowl of grapes sign (multiloculated appearance of mass with internal septations). On T1W images, SS demonstrates the split-fat sign on T1 (a thin rim of fat around mass due to intermuscular origin near neurovascular bundle).

Extra-skeletal myxoid chondrosarcoma
It is a rare malignant mesenchymal neoplasm with a haemorrhagic, multinodular appearance. It most commonly affects adults in their fifth and sixth decades with a slight male predominance. Patients often present with a slowly enlarging, deep-seated soft tissue mass, often accompanied by pain and tenderness. Tumours close to joints may restrict movement. Some tumours may mimic a haematoma. They have a high risk of local recurrence and metastasis, where they most commonly metastasis to the lungs. They can also metastasise to soft tissue and lymph nodes. However, they may have prolonged survival with metastases (10-year survival 70–88%). Treatment is by radical local excision and adjuvant radiotherapy.

Most lesions arise in the deep soft tissues of the proximal extremities and limb girdles, and the thigh is the most commonly affected site. However, lesions can also occur in the trunk and paraspinal (Figure 9.4A). The median size of lesions is 7 cm. They are well-defined soft tissue masses consisting of nodules of various sizes.

Figure 9.3: (A) Synovial sarcoma. AP radiograph of the pelvis (a) demonstrates amorphous calcification partially overlying the left proximal femur without any periosteal reaction. A coronal T1-weighted image (b) demonstrates a complex mass in the quadriceps muscles. A coronal fluid-sensitive fat-suppressed image (c) reveals a complex heterogenous mass which was subsequently proved to be synovial sarcoma on biopsy. (B) Synovial sarcoma. STIR short-axis (a) and long-axis (b) images show deep plantar soft tissue mass showing complex solid cystic appearances with fluid-haemorrhagic levels (curved arrows) and permeative infiltration of the second metatarsal shaft (straight arrow). Post-contrast short-axis (c) image shows enhancing soft tissue component (asterisk) and peripheral enhancing cystic components. Greyscale ultrasound image (d) shows biopsy through the solid component. (Image Courtesy of Dr. Harun Gupta.)

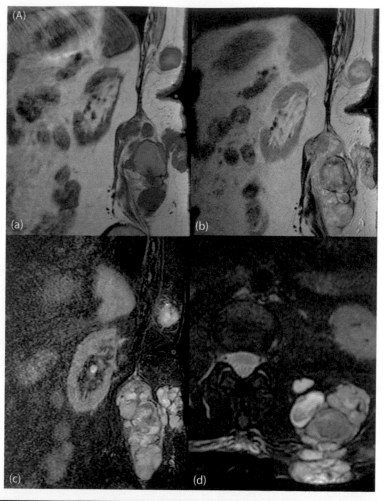

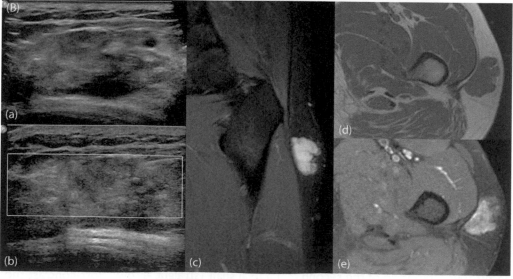

MRI features

MRI lesions are heterogeneously T1 isointense to muscle and commonly have internal haemorrhagic foci, manifesting as high T1 signal intensity. On T2W images, lesions are heterogeneously hyperintense to muscle and often contain regions of homogenous high signal necrosis or myxoid tissue. Fluid-fluid levels have also been reported. They display homogenous or heterogeneous (Figure 9.4B) contrast enhancement more intense at the periphery, which corresponds to increased cellularity. They may also exhibit an incomplete low-signal rim surrounding nodules.

UNDIFFERENTIATED SARCOMA

It includes undifferentiated spindle cell sarcoma and undifferentiated pleomorphic sarcoma (Figure 9.5). These entities have newly been merged into tumours of uncertain differentiation in the new WHO 2020 classification.

They are uncommon mesenchymal neoplasms that have no anatomical predisposition. They occur at all ages and with no gender predilection. Their aetiology is unknown; however, at least 25% of radiation-associated soft tissue sarcomas are undifferentiated.

Undifferentiated sarcomas have no pathognomonic imaging features. Instead, they present as a heterogeneous mass in the retroperitoneum and extremities.

Take-home points

- Tumours of uncertain differentiation are a challenging set of tumours to diagnose.
- Advances in molecular genetics are helping improve the diagnostic accuracy of some of these tumours.
- Additions, deletions and re-arrangement of key tumours as per the new WHO 2020 classification have been highlighted in the chapter. The radiologist needs to have an awareness of these changes.
- MRI is the imaging modality of choice for the characterisation of these lesions.

Figure 9.4: (A) Extra-skeletal myxoid chondrosarcoma. Sagittal T1-weighted image of the posterior abdominal wall (a) demonstrates a large multilobulated mass involving the inferior erector spinae musculature with extension into the subcutaneous tissues. There is a further smaller discrete mass of similar internal morphology in the subcutaneous tissues further cranially. T2 (b) and STIR (c) sagittal sequences demonstrate internal heterogenous appearances with fluid-fluid levels. Axial STIR images (d) demonstrate extension of the lesion from the erector spinae musculature through to the quadratus lumborum. (B) Extra-skeletal myxoid chondrosarcoma in a separate patient. Greyscale (a) and colour Doppler (b) ultrasound images show heterogeneous soft tissue mass lesion involving the left lateral thigh subcutaneous fat. Coronal STIR (c), axial T1-weighted (d) and post-contrast (e) images demonstrate heterogenous soft tissue mass lesion which shows intense and heterogenous enhancement. (Image Courtesy of Dr. Harun Gupta.)

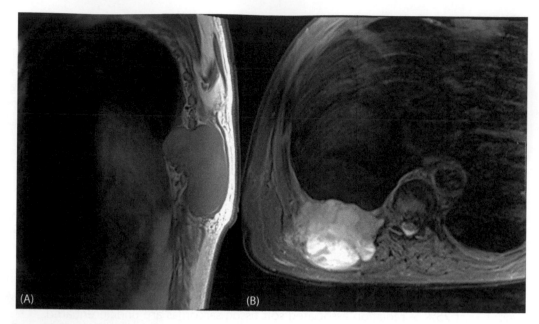

Figure 9.5: Undifferentiated pleomorphic sarcoma. Sagittal T1-weighted images (A) demonstrate a large mass in the right posterior chest wall. Axial T2 fat-suppressed sequences (B) reveal internal heterogenous fluid signal.

SUGGESTED READING

- Hussein, MAM, Cafarelli, FP, Paparella, MT, Rennie, WJ, Guglielmi, G. Phosphaturic mesenchymal tumors: Radiological aspects and suggested imaging pathway. Radiol Med. 2021;126(12):1609–1618. doi: 10.1007/s11547-021-01412-1.
- Kransdorf, MJ, Murphey, MD. Imaging of soft tissue tumors. Lippincott Williams & Wilkins; 2006.
- McCarville, MB, Muzzafar, S, Kao, SC, et al. Imaging features of alveolar soft-part sarcoma: A report from Children's Oncology Group Study ARST0332. Am J Roentgenol. 2014;203(6):1345–1352. doi:10.2214/AJR.14.12462.
- Mocellin, S. Soft tissue tumours: A practical and comprehensive guide to sarcomas and benign neoplasms. Springer; 2020.
- van Vliet, M, Kliffen, M, Krestin, GP, van Dijke, CF. Soft tissue sarcomas at a glance: Clinical, histological, and MR imaging features of malignant extremity soft tissue tumors. Eur Radiol. 2009;19(6):1499–1511. doi: 10.1007/s00330-008-1292-3.
- WHO Classification of Tumours Editorial Board. Soft tissue and bone tumours. Lyon (France): International Agency for Research on Cancer; 2020. (WHO classification of tumours series, 5th ed. Vol. 3). https://publications.iarc.fr/588 (Last accessed on 8 January 2022)

10 Other non-sarcomatous soft tissue tumours

Ramy Mansour,
Asimenia Mermekli,
Sandeep Singh Sidhu

INTRODUCTION

Non-sarcomatous soft tissue tumours are not uncommon and have not been specifically categorised in the recent World Health Organization (WHO) classification for soft tissue and bone, published in 2020 which is based on histological differentiation. These tumours include soft tissue carcinoma metastases, lymphomas, leukaemias, myelomas and large skin tumours. Soft tissue carcinoma metastases and haematologic malignancies can lead to significant morbidity and mortality.

SOFT TISSUE CARCINOMA METASTASES

Metastatic tumours presenting as masses in the muscles or subcutaneous tissue are relatively rare and can be the source of diagnostic confusion both clinically and pathologically. Several benign tumours and soft tissue sarcomas cannot be differentiated radiologically from soft tissue carcinoma metastases (STCM). These tumours may represent the initial manifestation of an occult primary. Therefore, histological recognition is very important. Most frequent symptoms are pain, palpable mass, swelling and cutaneous erythema.

The most common primary carcinoma causing soft tissue metastases are the lung (Figure 10.1) followed by the colon (Figure 10.2) and renal carcinoma. Thigh, gluteal, iliopsoas and paraspinal muscles are the most commonly affected sites. Metastases from lung cancer are localised frequently in upper (Figure 10.1) and lower extremities. Colorectal carcinomas metastasise often into the abdominal wall musculature. Urothelial carcinomas metastasise into the iliopsoas muscle and gastric cancer into the gluteal and lower extremities muscles. Psoas muscle metastatic disease is sometimes confused with psoas abscess or haematoma, both clinically and radiographically.

● Ultrasound

Soft tissue metastases appear as well-circumscribed hypoechoic and hypervascularised masses with no specific features (Figures 10.1 and 10.2).

DOI: 10.1201/9781003218722-10

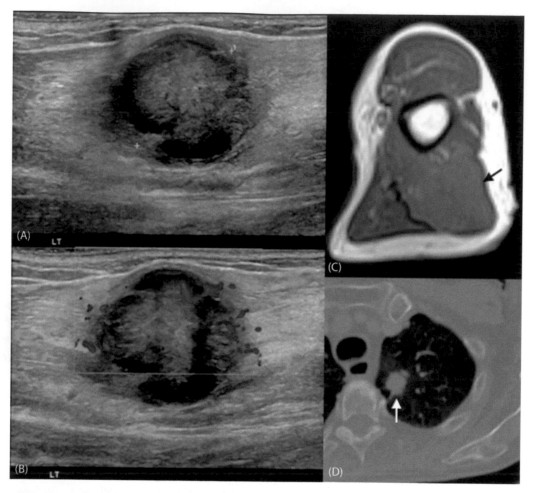

Figure 10.1: Intramuscular metastases in the lung cancer: Greyscale (A) ultrasound image demonstrates complex solid mass within the left triceps muscle which shows disorganised vascular flow on the colour Doppler (B) image. On MRI (C), the lesion appears isointense to the involving muscle (black arrow) which turn out to be a metastatic deposit on ultrasound-guided biopsy. The staging CT (D) demonstrates a spiculated mass lesion (white arrow) within the left upper lobe consistent with the primary tumour.

● *Computed tomography*

Computed tomography (CT) scan is not an ideal method for characterisation of soft tissue metastases. The most common appearance of soft tissue metastases on contrast-enhanced CT is that of an abscess-like intramuscular lesion with central low attenuation and rim enhancement. This appearance is more often seen in lung cancer. Metastases with multiple intramuscular calcifications are seen more often in gastric cancer. Calcification within soft tissue metastases can be confused with myositis ossificans, which is the formation of heterotopic ossification in large muscles post injury. Positron-emission tomography (PET)-CT may show avid tracer uptake.

● *Magnetic resonance imaging*

Magnetic resonance imaging (MRI) is the preferred technique for muscle and soft tissue assessment, even though MRI appearances of soft tissue metastasis are not specific and

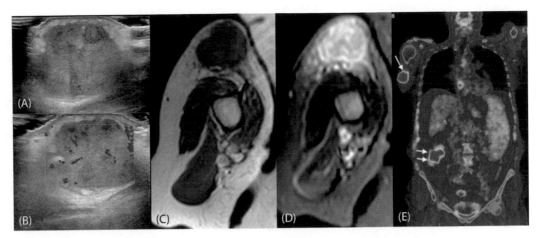

Figure 10.2: Subcutaneous metastatic deposit in the colon cancer: Greyscale (A) ultrasound image showing solid aggressive mass lesion in the anterior subcutaneous tissue of the right arm showing aggressive vascularity on colour Doppler (B) image. Corresponding T1-weighted (C) and STIR (D) images confirm aggressive nature of the disease without underlying muscle involvement. The lesion has confirmed to be a metastatic deposit from adenocarcinoma of the ascending colon seen on PET-CT (E). Please appreciate similar intensity of the radi-tracer uptake in the subcutaneous tissue (white arrow), anterior mediastinal lymph node and the primary lesion (double arrows).

metastases cannot be reliably distinguished from the primary soft tissue sarcoma. Lesions are of low or intermediate signal intensity compared to normal muscle on T1-weighted sequences and high signal intensity on T2-weighted sequences. Oedema of surrounding soft tissue is common. Erosion of the adjacent bone might rarely be observed on MRI. Most muscle metastases show marked heterogeneous enhancement. In addition, extensive peritumoral enhancement has been reported in some papers.

● Diffusion-weighted imaging

Diffusion-weighted imaging (DWI) is considered as a useful method in the assessment of tumour cellularity and can be used to monitor treatment responses. Some soft tissue metastases demonstrate moderate to high signal intensity on diffusion images and corresponding low or moderate apparent diffusion coefficient (ADC) values.

● Soft tissue melanoma and other skin carcinoma

The incidence of malignant melanoma has steadily been rising, with an average incidence ranging from 2 to 20% in most developed countries. Ultraviolet ray exposure is a known risk factor for melanoma. Diagnosis of malignant melanoma of the skin is based on clinical inspection and full-thickness biopsy. Primary melanoma most commonly arises from the skin, hence some patient present with a noticeable skin lesion. Melanoma may metastasise to the skin, soft tissues, lung, liver and brain. It can spread via both lymphatic and haematogenous routes, and is known for distant spread. Skin and subcutaneous lesions that occur within 2 cm of the primary tumour are known as satellite lesions, while those that occur beyond 2 cm are considered in-transit metastases.

Imaging plays an important role in staging and follow-up of patients with metastatic melanoma. CT scan is currently the most widely used technique for tumour staging, surveillance and assessment of therapeutic response, but ultrasound, MRI and PET-CT also plays an important role.

Melanoma may metastasise haematogenously to muscle. On CT, muscle metastases appear as soft tissue density lesions. On MRI, these lesions are intermediate/high signal intensity on T1-weighted images and mixed signal intensity containing high and low signal on T2-weighted images. High signal intensity of metastases on T1-weighted images has been noted particularly in malignant melanoma metastases because they contain melanin and may often bleed. On post-contrast imaging with CT or MRI, muscle metastases typically appear as enhancing nodules or masses relative to surrounding muscle. Metastatic disease can also present as solid nodules in the subcutaneous tissues (Figure 10.3).

PET-CT has better sensitivity than CT for the detection of melanoma soft tissue metastasis. Whole-body PET-CT is being commonly utilised. However, its limitations include spatial resolution (~6 mm), failure to detect non-FDG-avid metastases and lack of specificity.

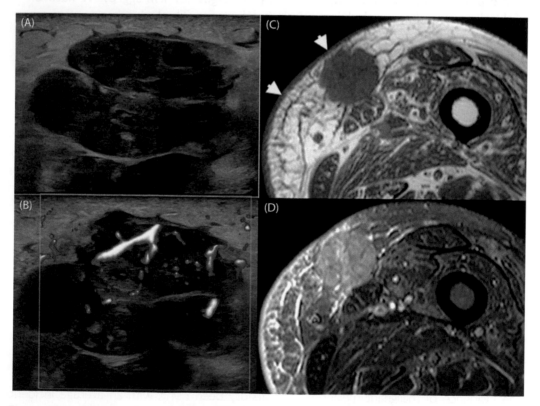

Figure 10.3: Metastatic melanoma: Greyscale (A) ultrasound image showing solid aggressive complex solid mass lesion in the subcutaneous tissue showing disorganised internal vascularity on colour Doppler (B) image. Corresponding T1-weighted (C) image shows hypointense lesion with increased signal on STIR (D) image with marked subcutaneous oedema and dermal thickening (yellow arrows). Metastatic melanoma demonstrates hyper- to hypointense signal on T1-weighted images depending upon the melanin content. (Image Courtesy of Dr. Harun Gupta.)

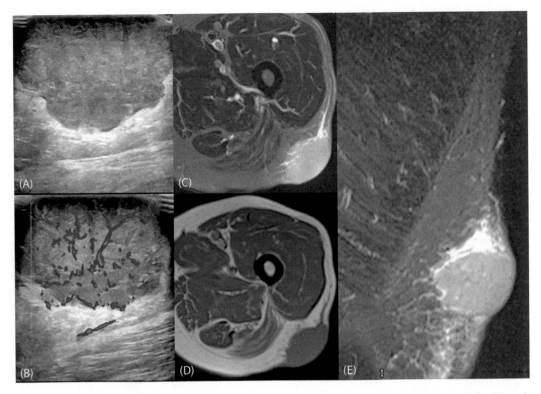

Figure 10.4: Merkel cell carcinoma: 77-years-old male patient presented with left gluteal mass lesion which appears solid on greyscale (A) ultrasound with disorganised vascularity (B). STIR axial (C) T1-weighted axial (D) and STIR coronal (E) images show solid subcutaneous lesion with marked dermal thickening and subcutaneous oedema. Imaging findings are non-specific. The lesion proved to be Merkel cell carcinoma on biopsy.

Merkel cell carcinoma (MCC) is a rare neuroendocrine skin cancer that occurs mainly in fair-skinned, elderly individuals (Figure 10.4). Globally, 80% of the tumours are initiated by Merkel cell polyoma virus (MCV) DNA integration into the cancer cells early in MCC development. MCC has an inherent capacity for early and aggressive local and systemic dissemination. Distant dissemination occurs in up to 40 to 50% of patients that develop visceral metastasis, particularly prevalent in the lungs, liver, bone and subcutaneous tissue.

SOFT TISSUE HAEMATOLOGIC MALIGNANCIES

Haematologic malignancies comprise clinically diverse diseases that can affect every organ system including the muscles and subcutaneous tissue. Haematologic malignancies include diseases such as Hodgkin's and non-Hodgkin's lymphoma (NHL), acute and chronic lympho-cytic and myelogenous leukaemia and multiple myeloma.

● *Lymphoma*

A soft tissue initial presentation of a lymphoproliferative neoplasm is a very rare occurrence accounting for approximately 0.1% of all lymphoid malignancies and 0.01% of all soft tissue tumours. Lymphoma should always be considered in extremity tumours thought to be sarcoma. The usual clinical symptoms are local swelling and pain or systemic symptoms such as fever, sweating and weight loss.

Commonly, soft parts are involved by direct extension from lymph nodes or other extranodal structures or by haematogenic dissemination. Soft tissue lymphomas generally present as painful subcutaneous masses in the thighs, trunk and lower limbs that are fixed on deep tissues and rapidly increase in size (Figures 10.5 and 10.6). Lymphomas can present as aggressive malignancies which spread across the anatomical boundaries without producing mass effect (Figure 10.7).

Muscular lymphoma is rare, representing up to 1.4% of all malignant lymphomas. It may occur as part of disseminated lymphoma, local extension from bone and lymphadenopathy or rarely

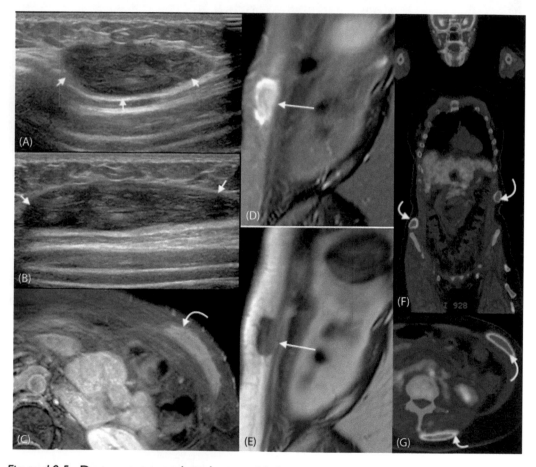

Figure 10.5: Deep cutaneous lymphoma with fascial involvement: Short-axis colour Doppler (A) and long-axis (B) ultrasound images showing solid mass lesion involving deep subcutaneous tissue of the anterior abdominal wall overlying the left external oblique muscle with splitting of underlying deep fascia (short arrows). There is visible mass effect over the muscle underneath the lesion but no frank invasion detected. It demonstrates hyperintense signal (arrow marked) on STIR axial (C) and sagittal (D) images and hypointense signal on T1-weighted signal (E). PET-CT fusion images in coronal (F) and axial (G) reformats show multiple deep subcutaneous areas of widespread disease showing marked radiotracer uptake (yellow curved arrows).

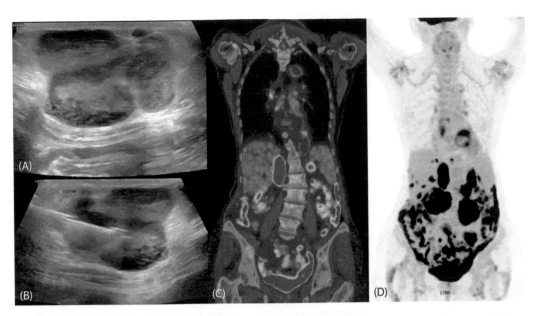

Figure 10.6: Extensive pelvic lymphomatous disease: Greyscale ultrasound image (A) demonstrates aggressive solid multiloculated lesion involving the deep soft tissue of the lower anterior abdominal wall. The ultrasound-guided biopsy (B) suggested lymphomatous tissue. The staging PET-CT depicts extensive infra-diaphragmatic nodal lymphomatous disease on fused coronal reconstructed (C) and PET (D) images.

primary muscular lymphoma (PML). PML is commonly due to NHL, including B cell, T cell and natural killer cell types. Clinical presentation may be acute or insidious or due to pain.

Muscular lymphoma is most common in the thigh and upper arm muscles. It may present as a focal mass or diffuse muscular infiltration. Ultrasonography features are non-specific and it appears as a heterogeneous, hypoechoic solid mass with irregular or poorly defined margins.

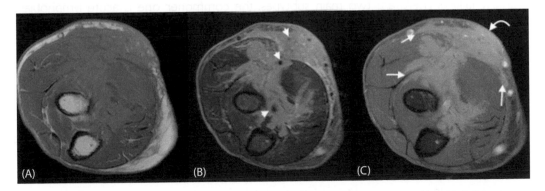

Figure 10.7: Infiltrative lymphoma: T1-weighted (A), STIR (B) and post-gadolinium T1-weighted fat-suppressed (C) axial images at the proximal forearm level demonstrate extensive soft tissue mass lesion showing multicompartmental muscular involvement. It shows permeative spread encasing the vessels (arrowheads), spreading along the fascial planes (arrows) and involvement to the subcutaneous tissue and the skin (curved arrow). Extensive spread along the neurovascular and fascial planes without mass effect on or destruction of the surrounding tissue is one of the characteristics of the lymphoma. (Image Courtesy of Dr. Harun Gupta.)

CT is also non-specific with tumour attenuation similar to or less than normal muscle and variable post-contrast enhancement. MRI is the most useful modality for assessment of muscular lymphoma and is the modality of choice for assessing local tumour infiltration.

On MRI, the lymphomatous skeletal muscle involvement can be suspected in cases of diffuse muscle enlargement with multicompartmental involvement, deep fascial involvement, the presence of traversing vessels in the lesion and skin thickening. Skeletal muscle lymphoma can exhibit peripheral thick bandlike enhancement or marginal septal enhancement in addition to the well-known finding of diffuse homogeneous contrast enhancement.

The most common MRI characteristics of a lymphomatous lesion are isointense to mildly hyperintense signal on T1-weighted scan (relative to muscle), intermediate signal between fat and muscle on T2-weighted scan, hyperintense signal on STIR and enhancement may be heterogeneous or homogenous. Planning of surgical tumour excisions is often based on the depth of infiltration found on MRI.

Current guidelines encourage the use of 18F-FDG PET/CT for primary staging of 18F-FDG-avid and potentially curable lymphomas (e.g. diffuse large B-cell lymphoma and Hodgkin's disease), particularly with regard to the 2007 revised response criteria that include the evaluation of tumour tissue metabolism. It also provides additional prognostic information.

18 F-FDG PET can determine a safe tumour-free surgical margin which is of great importance.

Ultimately tissue diagnosis is essential prior to commencement of treatment. However, in some instances, lymphoma may be missed on core biopsy, if there is a low index of suspicion.

● *Leukaemia*

Leukemias are the most common childhood cancer which arise from clonal proliferation of abnormal haematopoietic cells leading to disruption of normal marrow function and marrow failure. There are two main subtypes: the commoner one is acute lymphoblastic leukaemia (ALL) and acute myeloid leukaemia (AML). A small proportion may have chronic myeloid leukaemia (CML) and juvenile myelomonocytic leukaemia (JMML).

Extramedullary leukaemia refers to lesions that occur in any anatomical sites outside bone marrow. Granulocytic sarcoma (GS) (also known as myeloid sarcoma or chloroma) is a rare extramedullary manifestation which is commonly found in patients with AML. In most cases, it occurs after the diagnosis of the underlying malignancy and affects frequently the cutis and subcutis. Leukaemia cutis (LC) is a non-specific term used for cutaneous manifestations of any type of leukaemia. Legs are involved most commonly, followed by arms, back, chest, scalp and face.

Common manifestations are of anaemia, thrombocytopenia and neutropenia. These include pallor and fatigue, petechiae or purpura and infections. Lymphadenopathy, visceromegaly (hepatomegaly, splenomegaly, nephromegaly, enlargement of the pancreas) is a common finding. The diagnosis is confirmed by peripheral smear examination and/or bone marrow aspirate/biopsy.

Intramuscular deposits of leukaemia are very rare and generally are hypodense on CT scan and on MRI appear isointense to muscle on T1-weighted image and hyperintense on T2-weighted image. Soft tissue – skin (chloroma), subcutaneous tissue or muscles – deposits

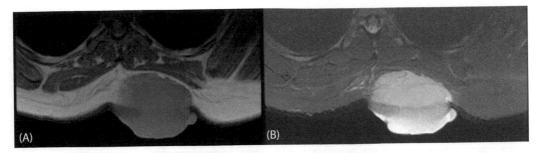

Figure 10.8: Cutaneous lymphoma: The patient previously treated for B-cell lymphoma presented with a solid mass involving the left paraspinal skin and subcutaneous fat showing hyperintense signal on T1-weighted (A) and STIR (B) images compared to underlying paraspinal muscles. (Image Courtesy of Dr. Harun Gupta.)

are not pathognomic on imaging and should be kept in differentials whilst evaluating a leukaemic patient with a newly developed soft tissue lump. Soft tissue leukaemia deposits may sometimes mimic cutaneous lymphoma (Figure 10.8) or primary skin tumours. Image-guided biopsy is usually required to confirm.

PET-CT significantly contributes to the diagnosis and treatment of different types of leukaemia, especially evaluation of extramedullary infiltration, monitoring relapses and assessment of the inflammatory activity associated with acute graft versus host disease.

A systematic approach is necessary for diagnosis. Radiologists should be aware of initial radiological manifestations of the disease, especially extramedullary involvement, in order to suspect the diagnosis of leukaemia in its early stage.

● *Multiple myeloma/plasmacytoma*

Extraosseous involvement of multiple myeloma has increased in the past several decades, possibly due in part to improved imaging detection and increased patient survival. Multiple myeloma is usually confined to the skeletal system although there may be mixed bone and soft tissue involvement with osseous lesions dominant. In a small number of instances, extraosseous lesions dominate with or without overt bone disease.

Extramedullary plasmacytomas (EMP) are rare, representing only 4% of all plasma cell neoplasms and arises from proliferations of monoclonal plasma cells. In primary form, these malignancies occur without other sites of plasma cell disease. Secondary extramedullary plasmacytomas occur in association with multiple myeloma and may be discovered during initial intramedullary disease or may occur during multiple myeloma relapse. In very rare instances, secondary EMPs have multifocal skeletal muscle and subcutaneous involvement.

Imaging characteristics for soft tissue myeloma are non-specific and can be similar to primary soft tissue sarcoma. However, the presence of soft tissue masses in patients with a known history of multiple myeloma should raise suspicion for extraosseous disease (Figure 10.9). Tissue biopsy can help to confirm suspicions in equivocal cases.

When suspicion of localised EMP is established, PET-CT or whole-body MRI should be considered to identify the full extent of the disease and for follow up post chemotherapy.

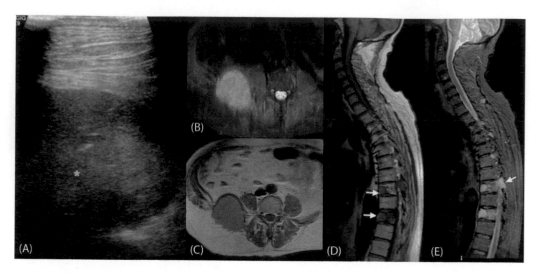

Figure 10.9: Soft tissue (muscular) myeloma deposit: Soft tissue mass (asterisk in A) involving the right quadratus lumborum muscle which shows corresponding STIR (B) and T1-weighted (C) signal (myeloma on biopsy). The MRI shows presence of a vertebral lesion. On further investigation, there were multifocal myeloma deposits in the whole-spine MRI on T1W (D) and STIR (E) sagittal images.

Take-home points

- We have provided a generalised overview on other non-sarcomatous soft tissue tumours which was not included in the WHO classification published in 2020.
- It includes soft tissue carcinoma metastases, lymphoma, leukaemia, multiple myeloma and skin cancer.
- There are no specific features on imaging for these tumours.
- Clinical history, histopathological and occasionally immunohistochemical analysis is essential for accurate diagnosis before commencement of treatment.

SUGGESTED READING

- Anderson, W. J., Doyle, L. A. (2021). Updates from the 2020 World Health Organization classification of soft tissue and bone tumours. *Histopathology*, 78(5). https://doi.org/10.1111/his.14265.
- Arun Visakh, R., Pratap, T., Mathew Babu, A., Abdul Jalal, M. J., Raja, S. (2018). In-transit metastasis of malignant melanoma. *Applied Radiology*, 47(11).
- Ginanni, B., Vallini, V., Marchetti, M., Lauretti, D. L., Cerri, F., Bozzi, E., Caramella, D., Bartolozzi, C. (2012). Usual and unusual imaging findings in metastatic melanoma (MM). *ECR 2012*.
- Laor, T. (2004). MR imaging of soft tissue tumors and tumor-like lesions. In *Pediatric Radiology* (Vol. 34, Issue 1). https://doi.org/10.1007/s00247-003-1086-3.
- Lim, C. Y., Ong, K. O. (2013). Imaging of musculoskeletal lymphoma. In *Cancer Imaging* (Vol. 13, Issue 4). https://doi.org/10.1102/1470-7330.2013.0036.
- Moore, R. D., Nelson, S. M., Cecava, N. D. (2020). Diffuse skeletal muscle extramedullary plasmacytomas: A rare case and review of the literature. *Skeletal Radiology*, 49(12): 2087–2093. doi: https://doi.org/10.1007/s00256-020-03514-9.
- Navarro, S. M., Matcuk, G. R., Patel, D. B., Skalski, M., White, E. A., Tomasian, A., Schein, A. J. (2017). Musculoskeletal imaging findings of hematologic malignancies. *Radiographics*, 37(3). https://doi.org/10.1148/rg.2017160133.
- Patnana, M., Bronstein, Y., Szklaruk, J., Bedi, D. G., Hwu, W. J., Gershenwald, J. E., et al. (2011). Multimethod imaging, staging, and spectrum of manifestations of metastatic melanoma. *Clinical Radiology*, 66(3).

- Surov, A., Hainz, M., Holzhausen, H. J., Arnold, D., Katzer, M., Schmidt, J., Spielmann, R. P., Behrmann, C. (2010). Skeletal muscle metastases: Primary tumours, prevalence, and radiological features. *European Radiology, 20*(3). https://doi.org/10.1007/s00330-009-1577-1.
- Tannenbaum, M. F., Noda, S., Cohen, S., Rissmiller, J. G., Golja, A. M., Schwartz, D. M. (2020). Imaging musculoskeletal manifestations of pediatric hematologic malignancies. *American Journal of Roentgenology,214*(2). https://doi.org/10.2214/AJR.19.21833.
- Thomas, R. Z., Dalal, I. B. (2018). Extraosseous multiple myeloma. *Applied Radiology, 47*(9). https://doi.org/10.1097/00000658-196911000-00019.

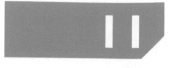

Soft tissue tumour mimics

Ganesh Hegde,
Karthikeyan P Iyengar,
Rajesh Botchu

INTRODUCTION

Soft tissue sarcomas are rare neoplasms; however, soft tissue "lumps and bumps" are frequently seen in day-to-day practice. Many non-neoplastic lesions mimic soft tissue tumours. A sound understanding of these lesions is essential for accurate diagnosis and for avoiding unnecessary interventional procedures. The list of conditions mimicking soft tissue tumours is exhaustive. This chapter aims to describe commonly encountered non-neoplastic soft tissue lesions.

Although most of the soft tissue tumours present as palpable masses, further characterisation of these lesions on clinical findings alone is challenging, and imaging is routinely performed for this purpose. Ultrasonography (US) and magnetic resonance imaging (MRI) are the modalities of choice due to their ability to characterise soft tissues. Radiographs and computed tomography (CT) scans are helpful in a few selected cases.

The different types of soft tissue tumour mimics covered in this chapter have been enumerated in Table 11.1.

Table 11.1: **Soft Tissue Tumour Mimics**

Post-traumatic lesions	Vascular lesions
Fat necrosis	Arteriovenous malformation
Haematoma	Aneurysm
Myositis ossificans	Pseudoaneurysm
Morel–Lavallee lesion	**Synovial abnormalities**
Calcific myonecrosis	Ganglion cyst
Muscle herniations	Synovial cyst
Infection	Bursae
Abscess	**Joint-based lesions**
Myositis	Gout
Inflammatory	Tumoural calcinosis
Rheumatoid nodule	**Miscellaneous**
Myositis	Epidermal inclusion cyst
	Accessory muscles
	Foreign body granuloma

DOI: 10.1201/9781003218722-11

POST-TRAUMATIC LESIONS

● *Fat necrosis*

A benign abnormality involving the subcutaneous fat. This condition is generally secondary to local trauma and presents as soft tissue masses with pain, mimicking a neoplasm. Other aetiologies such as exposure to cold, autoimmune disorders and vasculitis have also been implicated as a potential cause. In US, they may appear as a well-defined isoechoic lesion with hypoechoic peripheral halo or an ill-defined focus of hyperechoic subcutaneous fat with varying peripheral inflammatory changes. Rarely a central cystic or necrotic focus may be seen (Figure 11.1).

On MRI, it appears as a focus of fat with oedema and inflammatory changes on fluid-sensitive images. Occasionally, there may be a central necrotic component with peripheral contrast enhancement. A follow-up US imaging is helpful as they are known to reduce in size over time.

● *Haematoma*

They are commonly secondary to local direct trauma/contusion, sometimes a history of which may not be forthcoming or may be associated with muscle tears or avulsion injuries and can be seen in any tissue plane. They can occur following trivial trauma or spontaneously in patients on anticoagulants. In US, acute haematomas appear as poorly demarcated hyperechoic masses and, over time, become organised into more well-defined hypoechoic or mixed echoic lesions and may contain central liquefaction which can appear cystic. They are avascular and devoid of any vascular signal. On MRI, their appearance depends on the stage of the haematoma/haemoglobin. In general, areas of T1 hyperintensity and T2 hypointensity, often seen in the lesion's periphery, indicate the possibility of haematoma (Figure 11.2). A haematoma may mimic haemorrhagic soft tissue sarcoma. A painless, poorly defined mass (due to infiltrative margins) without a history of recent trauma, internal vascularity and progressive increase of the size on follow-up imaging should raise the suspicion of a neoplastic lesion.

Subacute to chronic muscle tears and avulsion injuries with associated organising haematoma may mimic a neoplasm. Awareness of these possibilities and their common sites with careful evaluation on MRI is often helpful inaccurate diagnosis.

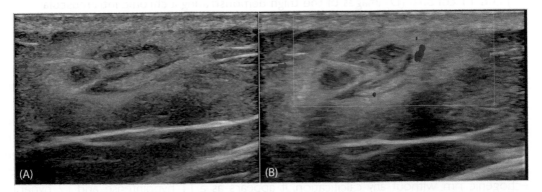

Figure 11.1: Subcutaneous fat necrosis: Greyscale ultrasound (A) and colour doppler images (B) show a heterogeneously hyperechoic hypovascular subcutaneous focus, consistent with subcutaneous fat necrosis.

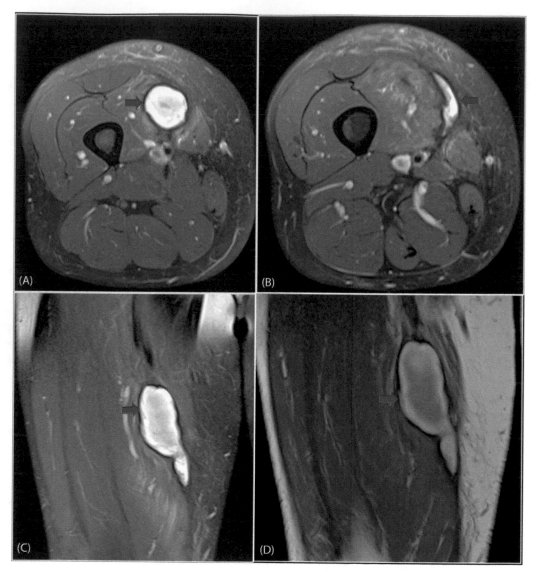

Figure 11.2: Haematoma: Proton density fat-saturated axial (A and B) and coronal (C) and T1 coronal (D) images of the thigh demonstrating a chronic intramuscular hematoma with extension in to the intermuscular plane.

● *Myositis ossificans*

A post-traumatic reparative process can simulate neoplasm that can be observed on both imaging and histopathology. They are more common in the anterior group of muscles in the thigh and arm. The imaging appearance of this lesion depends on the stage. Early lesions on plain radiograph and CT may appear as soft tissue swelling with no definite calcification. It is a hypoechoic lesion in the US with well-defined non-infiltrative borders and uninterrupted muscle fibres. It may show minimal internal vascularity. Some lesions may show peripheral echogenic rim without any calcification. It appears as a T1 hypointense and T2 hyperintense lesion with perilesional oedema on MRI. On T2 and post-contrast images, oedematous lesion with intact muscle fibres may demonstrate a striated appearance in the planes parallel to muscles and a checkerboard-like pattern due to hypointense muscle fibres within

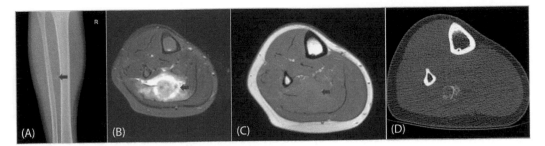

Figure 11.3: Myositis ossificans: Anteroposterior radiograph (A) of the leg shows an ill-defined calcified lesion in the mid-leg. Axial proton density fat-saturated (B) and T1 (C) MRI images show a heterogenous lesion with extensive surrounding oedema in the muscles of posterior aspect of the calf. Axial CT sections at the same level show a peripherally calcified lesion.

the oedematous lesion in the plane perpendicular to the muscle. As the lesion matures, it demonstrates calcification which extends from periphery to centre on all imaging modalities with a resolution of oedema and reduction of the overall size of the lesion (Figure 11.3).

● *Morel–Lavallee lesion*

These collections are located at the subcutaneous fat junction with deep fascia secondary to shearing injury following trauma. They are commonly located over bony prominences such as greater trochanter. Its appearance depends on the age of the contents, with acute lesions appearing more echogenic on the US with septations and echogenic fat globules. On MRI, they are primarily hyperintense on T2 with fat globules and haemorrhagic components appearing hyperintense on T1 and a hypointense fibrous capsule (Figure 11.4).

● *Muscle herniation*

These are protrusions of muscle through their fascial planes. Although commonly post-traumatic, they can also be congenital or following muscle hypertrophy. They are frequently encountered in lower limbs, with tibialis anterior being the commonest muscle involved. The

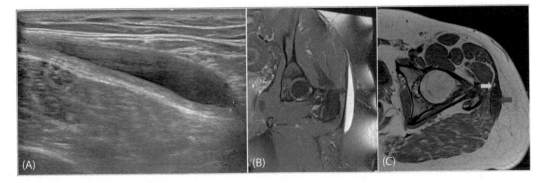

Figure 11.4: Morel–Lavallee lesion: Ultrasound (A) image demonstrating a linear collection at the junction of subcutaneous tissue with deep fascia, coronal proton density fat-saturated (B) and axial T1 (C) MRI images confirm this linear collection with a small peripheral fat lobule (yellow arrow).

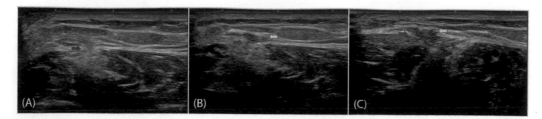

Figure 11.5: Muscle herniation: Greyscale ultrasound image at the level of mid-leg demonstrating a defect in the fascia covering the tibialis anterior (A). Further dynamic images (B and C) obtained with tibialis anterior in tension demonstrates herniating muscle fibres through the defect (yellow arrow).

dynamic US is the best imaging modality to diagnose as they can be seen herniating through the covering fascia when the involved muscle is put under tension/action (Figure 11.5).

● *Calcific myonecrosis*

Post-traumatic masses of dystrophic calcification characterise this condition. They are encountered almost exclusively in the lower limb, with the lower leg being the most commonly involved site. Radiographic appearances are characteristic of fusiform, large sheet of calcification in the involved entire muscle or compartment. On cross-sectional imaging, they appear as a fusiform lesion with a central cystic component with fluid calcium level. Blooming artefacts may be seen on MRI due to the presence of calcification (Figure 11.6).

INFECTIVE/INFLAMMATORY LESION

Musculoskeletal infections are not uncommon and can involve any tissue plane. When they are encountered with classical clinical features such as rapidly developing swelling, pain with fever and elevated inflammatory markers, the diagnosis is straightforward. However, on occasions, they are more indolent in their presentation and pose diagnostic challenges; this is particularly true with mycobacterial and fungal infections. In US, soft tissue abscesses appear as a hypoechoic collection with a heterochronic or echogenic rim and may contain internal echoes, debris and septation. They demonstrate mobile contents on compression and show peripheral Doppler signals with an avascular centre. On CT, they appear as peripheral rim enhancing lesions with surrounding stranding. CT is beneficial to identify air foci and useful when MRI is contraindicated. They appear heterogeneous on MRI. A T1 hyperintense periphery in the abscess cavity, also referred to as the Penumbra sign, is often characteristic of infection (Figure 11.7). Infective lesions demonstrate comparatively more perilesional inflammatory changes in comparison with neoplastic lesions. On contrast, the presence of thick irregular nodular enhancement favours a neoplasm. A central restriction of diffusion on diffusion-weighted images is more in favour of infection.

● *Myositis*

This could be infectious or inflammatory. In this condition, there is swelling of the muscle with oedema of the muscle fibres and sometimes mass-like appearance, which can mimic neoplasm. The ill-defined margin of the lesion, preservation of feathery pattern of the muscle, extensive perilesional oedema and presence of adjacent cellulitis favour infection over neoplasm (Figure 11.8).

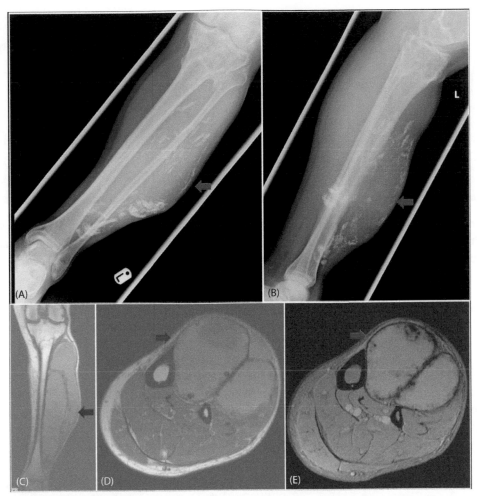

Figure 11.6: Calcific myonecrosis: Anteroposterior (A) and lateral (B) radiographs of the leg demonstrate a fusiform soft tissue lesion with peripheral plaque-like calcifications. Note evidence of previous healed fracture in the proximal tibia. Coronal T1W (C), axial T1W (D) and proton density fat-saturated (E) images of the leg demonstrate a large T1 iso- to hyperintense and PDFS hyperintense soft tissue mass.

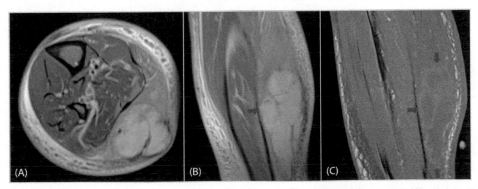

Figure 11.7: Abscess: Axial proton density fat-saturated (PDFS) axial (A), coronal (B) MRI images demonstrating a lobulated hyperintense collection in the muscular plane with extension in to the subcutaneous tissue. T1 coronal (C) image demonstrate a T1 hyperintense peripheral wall (red arrows) – Penumbra sign.

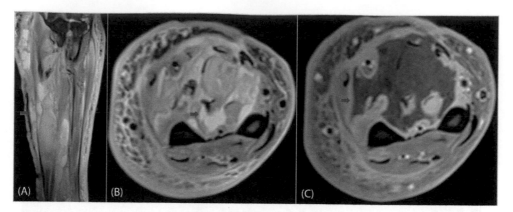

Figure 11.8: Pyomyositis: Proton density fat-saturated coronal (A) and axial (B) images show multiple pockets of collections involving the muscles of the anterior aspect of the forearm. T1 post-contrast fat-saturated axial (C) image demonstrates non-enhancing collection.

INFLAMMATORY LESIONS

● *Rheumatoid nodule*

They are the most frequent extra-skeletal manifestations of rheumatoid arthritis. Subcutaneous rheumatoid nodules occur at pressure points such as olecranon and heel pad. They appear as ill-defined hypoechoic subcutaneous lesions on the US with no internal vascularity. On MRI, they have variable appearances and generally are iso to hypointense on T1 and heterogeneously hyperintense on T2 without any significant contrast enhancement (Figure 11.9).

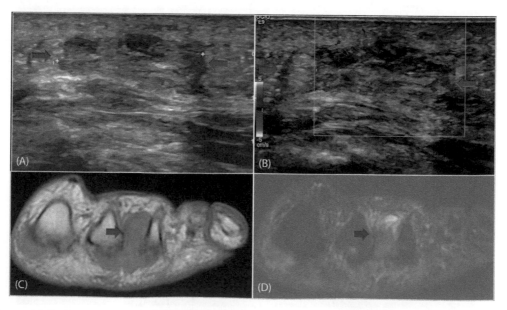

Figure 11.9: Rheumatoid nodule: Greyscale ultrasound (A) and Doppler images (B) demonstrate a hypoechoic, relatively hypovascular nodule in the second webspace. Axial T1W (C) and proton density fat-saturated (D) images of the foot demonstrate T1W iso- to hypointense and PDFS hypointense nodule in second webspace.

VASCULAR LESIONS

● *Arteriovenous malformation*

These are non-neoplastic hamartomas containing vascular channels in a fatty stroma. They are classified as slow-flow and high-flow vascular malformations depending upon flow dynamics and may be categorised as lymphatic, venous, capillary, arterial and mixed depending upon the vessel type. Most of the commonly encountered malformations are slow-flow malformations. On US, they appear as hypoechoic to anechoic, linear tubular structures with variable degrees of internal vascularity on Doppler. Phleboliths are characteristic findings and appear as echogenic foci with posterior acoustic shadowing. They can involve multiple tissue planes and may cross the compartments. On MRI, they are hyperintense on fluid-sensitive images and may show a variable amount of intralesional fat. Vascular flow voids and calcifications appear hypointense on MR images. MRI is often helpful in delineating the entire extent of the lesion, and mapping the feeding vessel and draining veins if they are present. The presence of phleboliths, intralesional fat and extension beyond tissue planes are useful findings to differentiate them from neoplastic lesions (Figure 11.10). Vascular lesions are described in detail in Chapter 8.

● *Aneurysms and pseudoaneurysms*

Aneurysms are dilatations of the artery containing all three arterial wall layers. Pseudoaneurysms are generally secondary to rupture of the arterial wall due to trauma

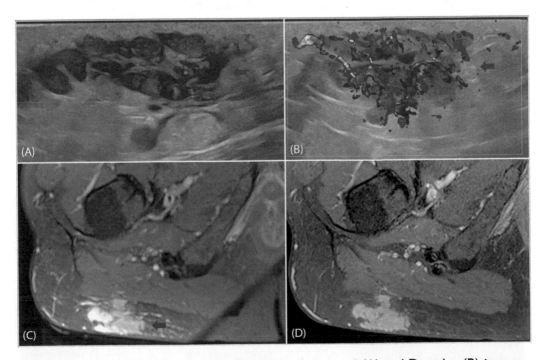

Figure 11.10: Vascular malformation: Greyscale ultrasound (A) and Doppler (B) images of the right buttock demonstrate a lobulated hypoechoic lesion with internal vascularity. Axial proton density fat-saturated (PDFS) (C) and T1 post-contrast fat-saturated (D) MRI images show a PDFS hyperintense avidly enhancing subcutaneous lesion.

or infection. Aneurysms are located along the course of an artery and continue with its lumen. Pseudoaneurysms are located eccentrically close to an artery and appear hypo to anechoic lobulated lesions on the US. On Doppler, they often demonstrate communication with the adjacent arterial lumen and also show a turbulent internal flow. They are often accompanied by a sizeable surrounding haematoma. CT angiography is the modality of choice for evaluating the extent, size and communication with the adjacent artery.

SYNOVIAL LESIONS

● *Ganglion cysts or synovial cysts*

They are cystic lesions containing myxoid material. Although not lined by synovium, they occur near the joint and tendon sheaths. They appear as unilocular cystic lesions on imaging with or without lobulations and show communication with adjacent joint or tendon sheath. When encountered with typical imaging findings, their diagnosis is often simple; however, they may demonstrate complex appearances with septations, debris and minimal internal vascularity, mimicking a neoplasm. Their location, close to a joint or a tendon sheath, predominantly cystic appearance, non-enhancing internal contents and extension or communication with the adjacent joint are helpful clues for their diagnosis.

Synovial cysts are synovial lined outpouchings commonly from a joint and contain synovial fluid. Baker's cyst is a classic example of a synovial cyst. Its typical location in the popliteal fossa, cystic appearance and communication with the joint cavity are often sufficient for the diagnosis; however, septation, synovial thickening, internal echoes and calcification/loose bodies may result in complex appearances mimicking a neoplasm. Apart from atypical appearances, synovial cysts can also create diagnostic dilemmas when encountered in atypical locations. A synovial cyst of the acromioclavicular joint, secondary to synovial fluid seeping through a chronic rotator cuff tear, may present as a pseudotumor (Figure 11.11). Similarly, a paralabral cyst or parameniscal cysts may occasionally create diagnostic dilemma. Their location close to a torn meniscus or labrum is a valuable clue for their diagnosis.

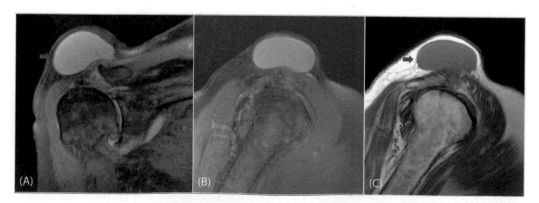

Figure 11.11: Ganglion: Proton density fat-saturated (PDFS) coronal (A), sagittal (B) and T1 sagittal (C) images showing ganglion (red arrow) in relation to ACJ with full thickness rotator cuff tear (Geyser phenomenon).

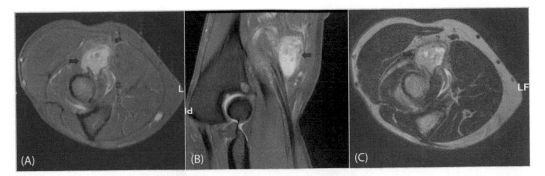

Figure 11.12: Bicipitoradial bursa mimicking a mass: Axial (A) and coronal (B) proton density fat-saturated images and axial (C) T2W MRI images of the elbow demonstrating a bicipitoradial bursa (red arrow) mimicking a soft tissue mass.

● *Bursitis*

Bursae are small fluid-filled synovial lined structures located around the joints, in-between the bone and tendon or over the pressure points. Bursitis is frequently encountered in daily practice and rarely confused with tumours. However, bursitis involving unique locations, such as bicipitoradial bursa (Figure 11.12) or obturator externus bursa, or when complicated by chronic synovitis, rice bodies, calcification and haemorrhage, may mimic neoplasm.

JOINT-BASED LESIONS

A few arthritic or metabolic conditions affecting the joint and surrounding soft tissues may result in lesions simulating a tumour.

● *Gout*

This condition is characterised by the deposition of monosodium urate crystals in joints and soft tissues. They rarely create diagnostic problems when they occur at classical locations with characteristic bone erosions. However, when tophaceous gout involves soft tissues at unusual locations, it can mimic a tumour. On radiographs, they appear as soft tissue swelling that may contain calcification foci. On US, tophi appear heterogeneously hyperechoic foci with calcifications. On MRI, they appear as iso- to hypointense on T1 and heterogenous or even hypointense on T2 due to calcifications (Figure 11.13). Dual-energy CT may help in definitive diagnosis by identifying the sodium monourate crystals in soft tissue tophi.

Similarly, soft tissue deposits may also be seen in CPPD disease and amyloidosis.

● *Tumoral calcinosis*

They are familial disorders characterised by the formation of large non-osseous calcific masses, mainly around the large joints. Other aetiologies such as end-stage renal disease, vitamin D toxicity, scleroderma have also been implicated. On radiographs, they appear as large amorphous multilobulated calcific periarticular masses containing septation. On CT scans, these calcified lesions show cystic areas, fluid-fluid or fluid calcium levels. On MRI,

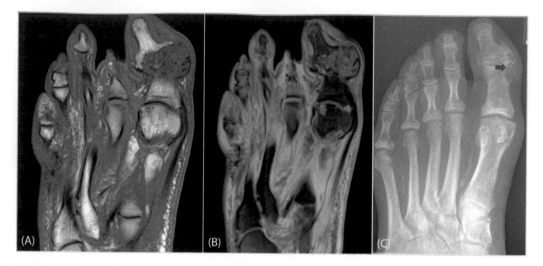

Figure 11.13: Tophaceous gout: T1 (A) and proton density fat-saturated (B) MRI images of the foot demonstrating a tophaceous gout deposit in the medial aspect of the interphalangeal joint of the great toe mimicking a soft tissue lesion. Corresponding radiograph (C) demonstrates characteristic gouty erosions in the base of the terminal phalanx and distal aspect of the middle phalanx (red arrow).

cystic areas appear hyperintense on T2 images and calcifications appear hypointense with perilesional oedema (Figure 11.14).

MISCELLANEOUS

● *Accessory muscles*

They are uncommon and often symptomatic. Sometimes, they may present with a pain-less visible swelling that mimics a soft tissue mass or produces symptoms due to nerve or vascular compression. They may be challenging to diagnose on imaging since they resemble normal skeletal muscle in all imaging modalities. On US, they may appear as an asymmetric thickening or relatively bulky area resembling normal muscle and are often challenging to diagnose since the entire extent may not be well visualised. On MRI, they are isointense to skeletal muscle on all the sequences. Accessory muscles have been

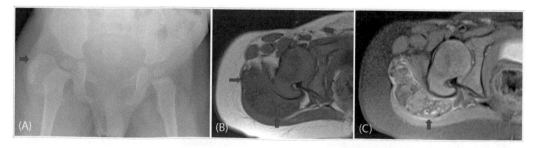

Figure 11.14: Tumoral calcinosis: Anteroposterior radiograph of the pelvis demonstrates a calcified soft tissue lesion in the lateral aspect of the right hip joint (A). Axial T1-weighted (B) and proton density fat-saturated (C) MRI images of the pelvis show a heterogeneous soft tissue mass in the posterolateral aspect of the hip consistent with tumoral calcinosis.

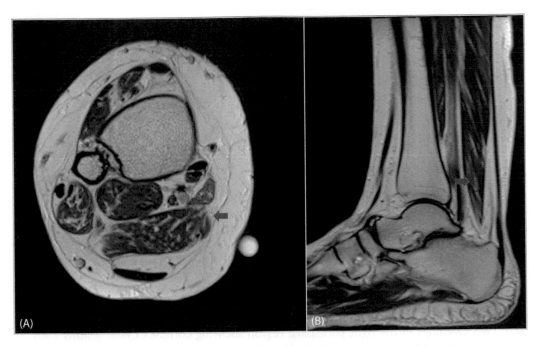

Figure 11.15: **Accessory muscle: T2 axial (A) and sagittal (B) images showing accessory soleus muscle presenting as a lump in the posteromedial ankle (note the skin marker at the site of described swelling).**

described in different locations. Awareness of this entity is essential for their diagnosis. If they are unilateral, comparison with the contralateral side may be helpful for identification (Figure 11.15).

● *Epidermal inclusion cyst*

They are non-neoplastic cysts and are the most commonly encountered cutaneous lesions. They can occur anywhere. They are thought to be secondary to the occlusion of pilosebaceous units of the skin. On US, they appear as heterogeneously hypoechoic cystic lesions. The presence of keratinous substances may give rise to internal echogenic foci. A linear punctum is often visible. They do not demonstrate internal vascularity (Figure 11.16). On MRI, they appear hyperintense on T2-weighted and hypointense on T1-weighted images and sometimes may show heterogeneous internal contents. A ruptured or infected cyst may demonstrate a more complex appearance with internal vascularity, surrounding oedema and irregular peripheral enhancement (Figure 11.17).

● *Pilomatricoma*

It is benign neoplasm seen at the junction of the dermis and subcutaneous fat. Pilomatricoma shows bimodal peak in the first and sixth decade and involves Caucasians and females commonly. The head and neck (most common) followed by upper extremities, trunk and lower extremities are involved sites. On ultrasound, they appear as ovoid complex masses at the junction of the dermis and subcutaneous fat with thinning of overlying skin. They show variable degree of calcification. Early lesions show punctate calcifications (Figure 11.18) with "target appearance" formed by intralesional hyperechoic epithelial cells and peripheral

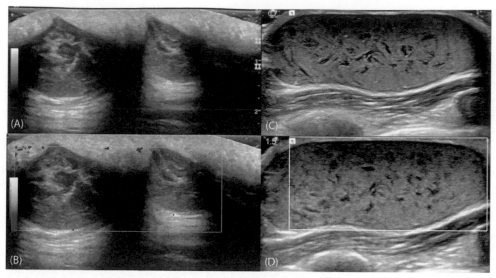

Figure 11.16: Typical ultrasound appearances of the epidermal inclusion cyst in two different patients: Greyscale (A) and colour Doppler (B) ultrasound images in a patient with two swellings in the right paraspinal region showing complex cystic lesions each with well-defined punctum through the dermis communicating to the exterior, marked through-transmission and lack of internal vascularity. A large sebaceous cyst in the right anterior chest wall (C and D) of more than 6 cm showing typical complex cystic appearances known as "pseudotestis appearance". (Image Courtesy of Dr Siddharth Thaker.)

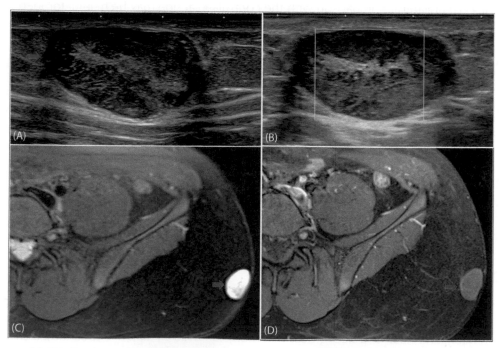

Figure 11.17: Epidermal inclusion cyst: Greyscale ultrasound (A) and colour Doppler (B) images demonstrate a heterogeneously hypoechoic lesion in the subcutaneous plane. Proton density fat-saturated (C) and post-contrast T1 fat-saturated axial (D) MRI image show a non-enhancing subcutaneous cystic lesion (red arrows).

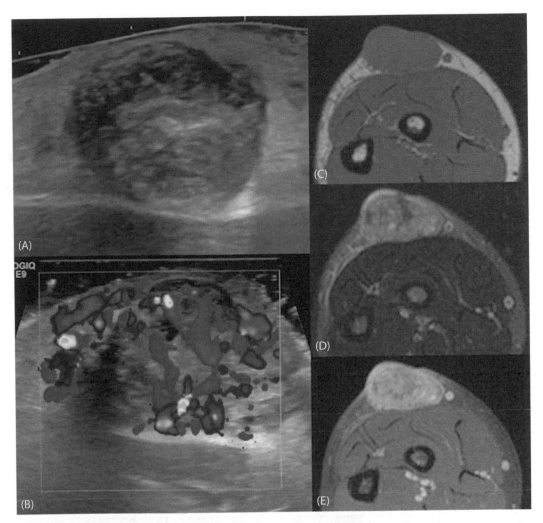

Figure 11.18: Pilomatricoma – early stage: Greyscale ultrasound (A) and colour Doppler (B) showing subdermal well-encapsulated, mixed echogenicity lesion showing marked internal vascularity. Corresponding MRI images showing homogenous mass lesion on T1-weighted (C) and heterogenous mass on STIR (D) images which shows intense variable enhancement (E) on post-contrast images. (Image Courtesy of Dr. Harun Gupta.)

fibrotic rim. More mature lesions show amorphous dense intralesional calcification with post-acoustic shadowing (Figure 11.19). Calcifications are better seen on radiographs and CT. On MRI, they appear homogenously hypo- to hyperintense on T1-weighted images and heterogenous on fat-suppressed water-sensitive images and following gadolinium administration. Surgical excision is the curative treatment for these lesions.

● *Tibial periosteal ganglion*

It is a rare, well-demarcated, smooth-walled, ganglion cyst arising from possible mucinous degeneration of the periosteum of the long bones. Most commonly seen involving the tibia near pes anserine tendons, other common sites include intercondylar region of the femur, metatarsal bones and the tarsal tunnel. It appears as an anechoic lesion with posterior acoustic enhancement, cortical remodelling and demonstrates a characteristic "mirror image

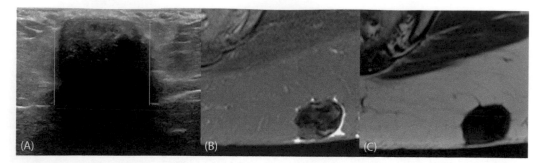

Figure 11.19: Pilomatricoma – matured: Greyscale ultrasound image (A) showing mature intralesional calcification casting a dense posterior acoustic shadow. STIR (B) and T1-weighted (C) images showing hypointense subdermal lesion with reactive soft tissue oedema. Proven pilomatricoma on excision biopsy. (Image Courtesy of Dr. Harun Gupta.)

artefact" at the bony cortex. There is lack on intralesional vascularity on Doppler imaging. MRI is the best modality to locate, characterise and follow up such evolving periosteal ganglion. It demonstrates typical features of a cyst (Figure 11.20) with homogenous T1-weighted signal depending upon its contents, uniform T2-weighted hyperintense signal and peripheral enhancement following gadolinium administration.

● *Foreign body granulomas*

A retained foreign body may incite a granulomatous reaction to form a foreign body granuloma which can resemble a mass. Ultrasound is the imaging modality of choice due to its high spatial resolution and ability to demonstrate a radiolucent foreign body. On US, foreign bodies appear as a linear echogenic structure with surrounding granulomatous inflammatory

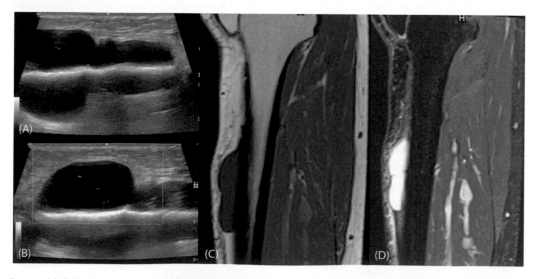

Figure 11.20: Tibial periosteal ganglion: Greyscale (A) and Doppler (B) ultrasound images show well-defined cystic lesion opposed to the tibial cortex with "mirror image artefact" and the lack of internal vascularity. T1-weighted (C) and T2-weighted fat-suppressed (D) sagittal images showing a cystic lesion elevating the tibial periosteum. (Image Courtesy of Dr. Harun Gupta.)

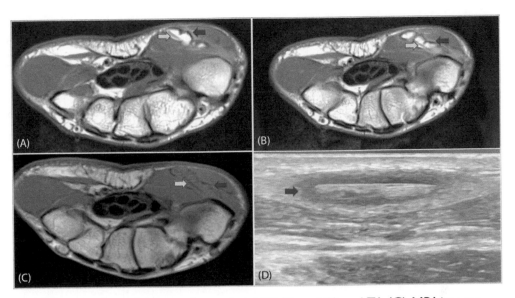

Figure 11.21: Foreign body granuloma: Axial T2 (A and B) and T1 (C) MRI images demonstrating a small collection in the thenar muscles of the hand appearing hyperintense on T2 and hypointense on T1 (with peripheral hypointense wall (red arrow). Linear hypointense foreign body seen in the centre (yellow arrow). Greyscale ultrasound image (D) demonstrating a subcutaneous linear echogenic foreign body with surrounding hypoechoic inflammatory changes (red arrow).

soft tissue appearing hypoechoic. They may show increased vascularity due to inflammation. On MRI, the foreign body is often hypointense on all the sequences, with surrounding inflammation appearing hyperintense on fluid-sensitive sequences. Diagnosis is straightforward if there is a history of recent penetrating injury and if a foreign body is demonstrable on imaging. In the absence of it, the inflammatory lesion may mimic neoplasm (Figure 11.21).

Take-home points

- Many non-neoplastic conditions mimic soft tissue tumours, and imaging is frequently needed to characterise them.
- US and MRI are primary imaging modalities used to characterise soft tissue lesions.
- Some of the tumour mimics, such as infection, may present with systemic symptoms, and correlation with clinical and laboratory findings is often helpful.
- A recent history of trauma or anticoagulant use helps diagnose a haematoma.
- Follow-up imaging may help in the definitive diagnosis of some of these mimics, such as haematoma and myositis.
- Some of these lesions may still remain indeterminate after clinical and imaging assessment and may need a biopsy for definitive management.

SUGGESTED READING

- Coran, A, Orsatti, G, Crimì, F, Rastrelli, M, Maggio, AD, Ponzoni, A, et al. Non lipomatous benign lesions mimicking soft-tissue sarcomas: A pictorial essay. In Vivo. 2018;32:221–229. Available from: https://iv.iiarjournals.org/content/32/2/221
- McKenzie, G, Raby, N, Ritchie, D. Non-neoplastic soft-tissue masses. Br J Radiol. 2009;82:775–785. Available from: http://www.birpublications.org/doi/10.1259/bjr/17870414

- Paramesparan, K, Shah, A, Rennie, WJ. Guide to pseudotumours and soft tissue tumour mimics. Orthop Trauma. 2017;31:204–215. Available from: https://linkinghub.elsevier.com/retrieve/pii/S1877132717300362
- Shah, A, Paramesparan, K, Robinson, P, Rennie, WJ. Non-neoplastic soft tissue tumors and tumor-like lesions. Semin Musculoskelet Radiol. 2020;24:645–666. Available from: http://www.thieme-connect.de/DOI/DOI?10.1055/s-0040-1713606
- Stacy, GS, Kapur, A. Mimics of bone and soft tissue neoplasms. Radiol Clin N. 2011;49:1261–1286.
- Wu, JS, Hochman, MG. Soft-tissue tumors and tumorlike lesions: A systematic imaging approach. Radiology. 2009;253:297–316. Available from: http://pubs.rsna.org/doi/10.1148/radiol.2532081199

12 Biopsy of soft tissue tumours

Siddharth Thaker, Harun Gupta

INTRODUCTION

The biopsy is the procedure of choice for the definitive diagnosis of soft tissue lesions. Not all soft tissue lesions require biopsy. For example, some benign lesions such as cysts/ ganglions and small superficial typical benign lipomas do not need further imaging or treatment. Typically, the indeterminate or overtly aggressive lesions on imaging require biopsy. Open, punch or excision biopsies are usually performed by the sarcoma surgeons, whereas radiologists perform biopsies using imaging guidance.

The following questions must be considered before biopsy:

- Is the biopsy indicated?
- How should the biopsy be performed? What is the best approach?
- Should the biopsy be performed by a musculoskeletal radiologist or a sarcoma surgeon?
- How will the patient be managed after the biopsy results?

In this chapter, we will review several essential points about image-guided biopsy. They are performed using ultrasound or CT scan guidance. General principles remain the same for all image-guided biopsies.

WHY BIOPSY?

Despite advances in imaging, a significant proportion of soft tissue lesions remain indeterminate on imaging. Definitive diagnosis on imaging alone is only possible in one-fourth to one-third of soft tissue lesions. Even when there are overt features of the aggressive nature of the lesion, a biopsy is indicated to identify histological type and grade and immunophenotyping to help in further management.

TYPES OF BIOPSIES

● Punch biopsy

It is usually reserved for dermal-based superficial lesions and performed by either a surgical team or dermatologists.

DOI: 10.1201/9781003218722-12

● *Excision biopsy*

It is performed for smaller superficial lesions, typically less than 2 cm, without any deep extension. There is no definite cut-off for the smallest dimension. The sarcoma team usually weighs risks versus benefits for image-guided biopsy in small lesions. The choice also depends upon the hospital logistics as a smaller-throw (e.g. 1 cm) needle may be available. If required, the radiologist may perform an image-guided biopsy for the smaller lesion.

● *Core biopsy*

It is the procedure of choice for larger, indeterminate or aggressive appearing soft tissue lesions and can be safely performed under imaging guidance.

● *Open biopsy*

The sarcoma surgeons usually perform such biopsies following a multidisciplinary team (MDT) meeting discussion in cases where other forms of biopsies can be challenging or less likely to be tolerated by the patient, such as neural lesions in line of major nerves.

● *FNAC*

We do not recommend it for soft tissue lesions due to its low diagnostic yield.

● *Aspiration*

Only cytological analysis can be done in cases with significant fluid content in the lesion. Aspiration can be considered if there is significant fluid content in the lesion. Aspiration may be performed for ganglia and symptomatic Baker's cysts (Figure 12.1).

BIOPSY

● *Preprocedural assessment*

One should review patient's current and past medical history and medication history. It is imperative to check whether the patient is on anticoagulation (such as warfarin or newer

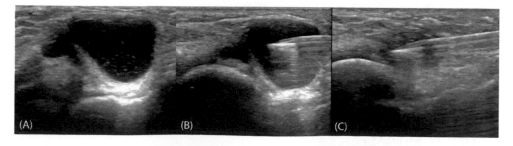

Figure 12.1: US-guided aspiration of the dorsal wrist ganglion. Three sequential greyscale ultrasound images showing dorsal wrist ganglion (A), aspiration using a 21-gauge needle (B), and note near complete collapse of the ganglion (C). Depending upon the contents of the ganglia, fenestration and steroid injection can be performed if required. The patient should be made aware that such ganglia can sometimes recur.

Table 12.1: Soft Tissue Lesion Biopsy Anticoagulation Guidance

If the lesion is **Superficial or immediate subfascial** <ins>and</ins> **Lack of significant vascularity**	• No action necessary for most medications • Still use 16G biopsy needle for the biopsy **If the patient is on warfarin, check INR is not beyond the therapeutic range for the patient**
If the lesion is **Deep and/or markedly hypervascular**	• Aspirin – Continue medication • Clopidogrel – Continue medication • Warfarin – Target INR is less than or equal to 3 (follow the local guidelines and discuss with haematologist if needed) • Low-molecular-weight heparin (LMWH) in a therapeutic dose – Hold one dose before the biopsy. If it cannot be stopped due to underlying reasons for anticoagulation, then this should be discussed with clinicians

direct oral agents like rivoroxaban, dabigatran, apixaban) or anti-platelet (such as clopidogrel) treatment.

It is essential to adhere to the local guidelines about anticoagulation during the ultrasound-guided biopsy. Although such policies vary between different centres, we have provided a model guideline for the readers (Table 12.1) to refer to. When uncertain, we recommend direct discussion with the sarcoma team to assess the risk-verses-benefit ratio from the potential discontinuation of the anticoagulants.

● *Fundamental principles of preprocedural image review*

A careful review of all available prior imaging should be done to plan the biopsy approach. We recommend reviewing cross-sectional imaging to ascertain the shortest and the safest biopsy approach.

One should avoid going through multiple compartments and neurovascular structures (Figure 12.2).

We also recommend avoiding areas of necrosis and haemorrhage and targeting the solid and enhancing areas if contrast-enhanced imaging is available. Such regions can provide the highest diagnostic yield preventing the need for repeat biopsies (Figure 12.3). Sometimes, the tumour may demonstrate extensive necrosis and solid components requiring a combined procedure – aspiration for the necrosed portion and the biopsy of the solid component (Figure 12.4).

● *Tract seeding*

Many sarcoma surgeons prefer site-specific surgical access to approach suspected neoplastic lesions. The biopsy approach must be discussed in the sarcoma MDT with the named sarcoma surgeon before agreeing to image-guided sampling as the surgeon might need to

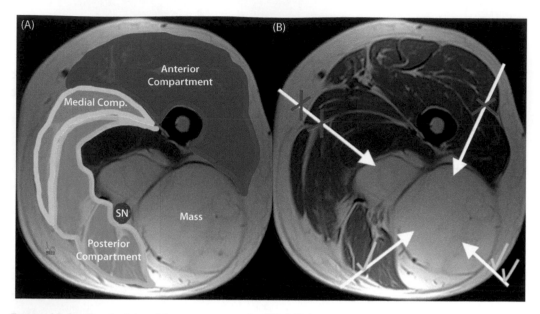

Figure 12.2: Optimising biopsy approach. (A) MRI image showing an aggressive predominantly fatty mass lesion in the posterior compartment of the left thigh. All compartments and sciatic nerves (SN) are colour coded to understand the compartmental anatomy better. (B) Biopsy approaches through the anterior and medial compartment would be suboptimal as they involve multiple compartments. Whereas the posterior compartment approach directly through the subcutaneous fat is the best approach as it is only via single subcutaneous compartment.

excise the biopsy track should the lesion demonstrate high histological grade. It is a good practice to mark a provisional biopsy approach on the cross-sectional imaging and saving such "key" images for preprocedural review (Figure 12.5).

A typical image-guided biopsy involves multiple passes into the lesion and can lead to breach of the tumour capsule numerous times. The authors often use a coaxial technique to minimise the risk of biopsy tract seeding in suspected deep-seated high-grade sarcomas (Figure 12.6).

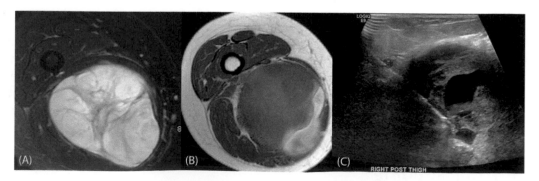

Figure 12.3: High-yield tumoral area target for biopsy. (A and B) MRI showing an aggressive mass with necrotic and solid areas. One of the solid areas was targeted (C) under US guidance for optimum diagnostic yield.

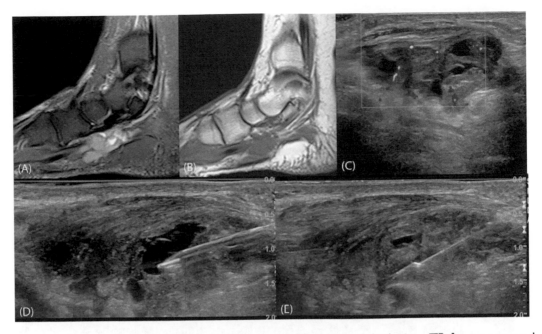

Figure 12.4: Modifying the technique according to the need of the lesion. T2-fat-suppressed (A) and T1-weighted (B) images show an aggressive soft tissue mass lesion within the deep medial aspect of mid-foot. The lesion appears solid-cystic with disorganised vascularity in colour Doppler (C) image. Aspiration (D) and biopsy (E) were performed in the same lesion. Histological diagnosis – synovial sarcoma.

● *Set-up and consenting*

All image-guided biopsies must be performed in the dedicated hospital setup. Informed consent is mandatory before the biopsy. One should take ample time to discuss the procedure with the patient and provide the reason for the biopsy and how long the results usually take to help allay the patient's anxiety. Where possible, written informed consent should be obtained documenting risks of bleeding, bruising, pain, infection, a non-diagnostic sample and the need to repeat the procedure.

● *Procedure*

Once consented, one should methodically approach the biopsy. Aseptic precautions are required using the site-cleaning solution, sterile probe cover and sterile ultrasound gel. The choice of site-cleaning solution depends upon the choice of the operator and hospital. We use 3-ml cutaneous solution containing chlorhexidine gluconate (20 mg/ml) and isopropyl alcohol (0.70 ml/ml). A brief diagnostic ultrasound should be performed to reassess the lesion for interval changes that may have happened since the initial planning scan. Optimal local analgesia using 1% lignocaine to the skin and soft tissue surrounding is generally sufficient for the biopsy. Care should be taken not to infiltrate the lesion with lignocaine beyond its capsule.

The choice of biopsy needles depends upon the operator, the lesion and the hospital logistics. The authors predominantly use a 16-gauge tru-cut side-cutting biopsy needle with a 2-cm throw. Needles with small throw and end-cutting biopsy needles are also available

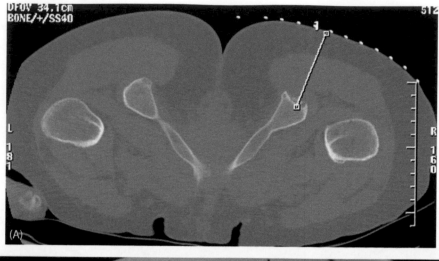

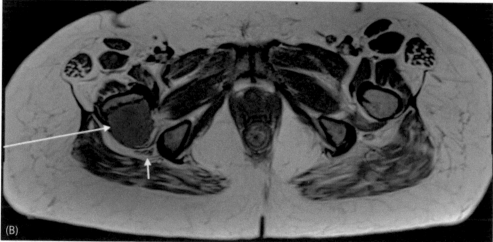

Figure 12.5: Biopsy planning in two different patients. (A) Non-contrast axial CT image in a patient with a history of breast carcinoma showing increased radiotracer uptake at the ischial tuberosity. Appreciate the marked position, which is subsequently used for needle placement. (B) T2-weighted axial image in a different patient with a history of papillary thyroid carcinoma showing isolated bone lesion in the right lesser trochanter. The posterolateral incision was planned for surgery. Therefore, the biopsy was performed using a similar path (white arrow) and the biopsy tract was excised during the definitive excision of the lesion. Note the position of the right sciatic nerve (yellow arrow).

(Figure 12.7). A smaller 18-gauge biopsy needle may be necessary if the lesion is in the superficial or challenging anatomical location (e.g. in the upper limb) or the patient may not be able to tolerate a wider bore needle (e.g. suspected neural lesion). A few centres use thicker 14-gauge core biopsy needles. An optimum number of the core samples is another controversial question one may face. We routinely obtain three cores as long as the patient remains comfortable. Sometimes, we may conclude the procedure if the patient is in significant distress or discomfort after obtaining two cores. If samples appear grossly non-diagnostic, for example, fragmented or liquid cores, one can make more attempts to get good cores if the patient can tolerate the procedure. However, this is an uncommon occurrence

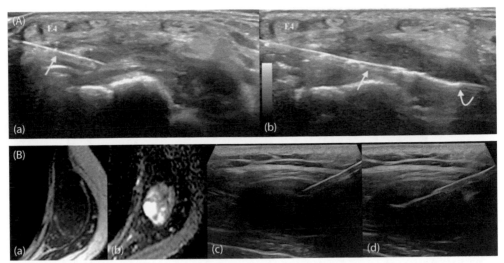

Figure 12.6: (A) Coaxial biopsy needle technique: (a) Greyscale ultrasound image showing an 18-gauge introducer needle placed within the wrist joint for synovial biopsy using a dorsal approach between the fourth and fifth extensor compartment tendons and (b) the biopsy is taken multiple times preventing the need of the wrist capsule penetration during each attempt. The method reduces the risks of capsule, tendon and neurovascular bundle injuries during biopsies of small joints. (B) Coaxial biopsy needle technique: (a) T1-weighted and (b) STIR images showing deep aggressive soft tissue mass lesion involving the left lateral chest wall musculature in serratus anterior. Greyscale image (c) showing placement of a 15-gauge penetrator needle within the lesion followed by samples taken by a biopsy needle (d). Multiple core samples can be taken by changing the direction or angle of the penetrator needle. It prevents repetitive tumour capsule penetration and track seeding.

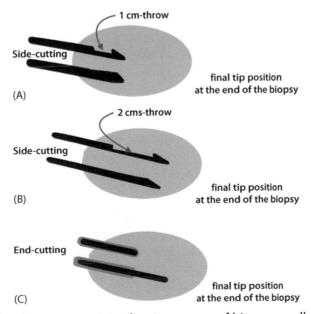

Figure 12.7: Graphical representation of various types of biopsy needles. (A) Side-cutting needle with a short 1-cm throw, (B) a long 2-cm throw and (C) an end-cutting needle. Note that the end-cutting needle advances from the final position of the tip during the throw, whereas the tip of the side-cutting needle marks the final position till which the needle will advance when "fired".

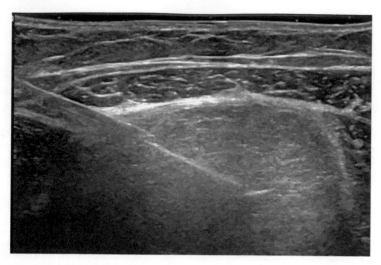

Figure 12.8: Storing biopsy images for future review and medico-legal purposes. Greyscale ultrasound image showing the intralesional position of the entire sampling portion of the biopsy needle in the suspected fatty lesion. Such an image would help indicate the appropriate biopsy technique should discrepancy arise between the histological grades of the biopsy sample and surgical specimen.

in authors' experience. The biopsy practice may differ amongst various centres; therefore, it is essential to adhere to local and regional guidelines.

Saving ultrasound images demonstrating optimal biopsy needle placement under ultrasound guidance is also an example of good practice (Figure 12.8). It may be helpful in cases where there is a discrepancy between radiological appearances and pathological findings.

Core biopsy samples are usually stored in a sterile container containing a fixative solution. A universal microbiological container may also be used if the infection is suspected. All samples should be correctly marked using the patient-specific identifiers and sent to the histopathology department via an agreed channel.

● *Postprocedural assessment and discharge*

Most of the biopsy procedures are uneventful, and the patient can be discharged safely after a 30-minute observation. We routinely provide an information leaflet containing a dedicated helpline number should the patient have further questions regarding the procedure and follow up.

Most common intra- and immediate postprocedural complications include bleeding and vasovagal syncope. Most postprocedural bleeds can easily be treated with pressure over the biopsy site. Uncontrolled bleeding is rare following percutaneous ultrasound-guided biopsy. Vasovagal syncope is common, especially in anxious patients. The majority of vasovagal symptoms are treated with conservative measures.

● *Follow-up MDT discussion*

Sarcoma pathologists usually rely upon numerous histological and immunochemical staining and cytogenetic analysis to determine the histological type, grade and overall grade of the tumour. The sarcoma team must discuss all patients undergoing ultrasound-guided biopsies to determine further management strategies.

As described earlier, patients with benign tumours can be safely discharged, followed up or removed depending upon the patient's preference. Locally aggressive tumours with limited locoregional spread may be treated by wide local excision, local radiotherapy or novel isolated limb perfusion chemotherapy. Malignant tumours on histology require a staging CT scan to exclude distant metastases. Such tumours may require aggressive treatment regimens, including limb sacrificing or preserving surgeries, radiotherapy and systemic chemotherapy to achieve a better prognosis.

CONCLUSION

An image-guided biopsy requires multidisciplinary discussion, a careful review of all imaging and strategic planning before attempting the procedure. Pre- and postprocedural sarcoma MDT discussion is essential to achieve optimum management of the biopsied soft tissue tumour.

Take-home points

- The sarcoma multidisciplinary team meeting must discuss soft tissue tumours requiring image-guided biopsy.
- One should use a methodical approach during the biopsy, including pre-procedural assessment, consent, good infection control, appropriate sampling and post-procedural sample processing whilst keeping the patient's comfort in the centre.
- Ideal preprocedural assessment includes careful review of clinical notes, all relevant imaging and patient-specific factors, including blood parameters.
- A quick ultrasound reassessment before the biopsy is essential to plan a safe and effective approach. It also helps select the region with the highest diagnostic yield and avoid neurovascular structures.
- Immediate postprocedural complications are uncommon and most of the complications can be managed conservatively.

SUGGESTED READING

- Bancroft, LW, Peterson, JJ, Kransdorf, MJ, Berquist, TH, O'Connor, MI. Compartmental anatomy relevant to biopsy planning. Semin Musculoskelet Radiol. 2007 Mar;11(01):016–027.
- Filippiadis, DK, Charalampopoulos, G, Mazioti, A, Keramida, K, Kelekis, A. Bone and soft-tissue biopsies: What you need to know. Semin Musculoskelet Radiol. 2018 Oct;35(04):215–220. Thieme Medical Publishers.
- Foremny, GB, Pretell-Mazzini, J, Jose, J, Subhawong, TK. Risk of bleeding associated with interventional musculoskeletal radiology procedures. A comprehensive review of the literature. Skelet Radiol. 2015 May;44(5):619–627.

13 Histopathology of soft tissue lesions

Sara Edward

INTRODUCTION

Soft tissue lesions include a large cohort of benign and malignant lesions arising from a variety of anatomical locations and tissue types.

Clinical history in terms of current and past lesions should be ascertained before and during the radiological assessment of any lesion.

Radiological assessment of the plane and location of the lesion plays a crucial role in the evaluation and final diagnosis of soft tissue lesions. This is particularly important in terms of the relationship of the lesion in question to the surrounding structures especially bone.

BIOPSIES

Particular attention should be paid, as far as possible, to obtain biopsies from viable tissue. This is important when needle core biopsies are performed on:

1 Cysts
2 Blood filled areas
3 Myxoid areas
4 Tumours with areas of necrosis

Special attention should also be paid to avoid structures which are normal to the site such as skeletal muscle and adipose tissue.

HISTOPATHOLOGY OF BIOPSIES AND RESECTED SPECIMENS

All specimens should be transported to the pathology department in an adequate amount of 10% formaldehyde (formalin), accompanied by the correct request form with adequate clinical and radiological information.

Clinical and radiological information is crucial in the microscopic assessment of the lesions and helps avoiding delays and correct interpretation.

The biopsies and resected specimens are evaluated using light microscopy, immunohistochemical stains and molecular techniques such as fluorescent in-situ hybridisation, mutational analysis and RNA fusion panel studies. Some tumours such as pleomorphic and dedifferentiated high-grade lesions may pose diagnostic dilemma in their final diagnosis where radiological input is vital to narrow down differentials.

DOI: 10.1201/9781003218722-13

Following the histopathological assessments, cases are discussed at multidisciplinary team meetings (MDTM) for correlation with clinical, radiological and pathological features and appropriate management strategies are decided.

There will be occasions of discrepancy between image-guided biopsies and resected specimens. The following may be the points of discrepancy in the diagnosis:

1 Benign vs. malignant
2 Neoplastic vs. inflammatory
3 Lesion vs. normal tissue
4 Final grade of the lesion (sometimes different parts of the lesion show different histological grades depending on criteria mentioned below. Therefore, percutaneous biopsy samples may not be representative of the final diagnosis)

MICROSCOPY OF SOFT TISSUE TUMOURS

Light microscopic evaluation is the first step in the pathological assessment of tumours. The current classification followed is the WHO classification 2020 of soft tissue tumours.

The cell types forming soft tissue tumours are:

- Adipocytes.
- Smooth muscle cells.
- Neural cells.
- Myofibroblasts.
- Small blue cells.
- Pleomorphic spindle cells NOS.
- Cells of uncertain histogenesis.
- Lipomas and liposarcomas (usual and myxoid liposarcomas) are formed of adipocytes.
- Leiomyomas and leiomyosarcomas are formed of smooth muscle cells.
- Neurofibromas, schwannomas and malignant peripheral nerve sheath tumours (MPNST) are formed of neural cells.
- Fibromas and myxofibrosarcomas are formed of myofibroblasts.
- Ewing's sarcoma is formed of small blue cell tumours.
- Synovial sarcoma and solitary fibrous tumours are formed of cells of uncertain histogenesis.
- Pleomorphic spindle cell sarcoma is a category of tumours with no definitive immunohistochemical or molecular features.

GRADING OF SOFT TISSUE TUMOURS

The internationally approved grading system is the **FNCLCC** (Federation Nationale des Centers de Lutte Contre le Cancer) grading system.

This is based on:

- Tumour differentiation: scores 1–3
- Mitotic activity (0–9 = score 1, 10–19 = score 2, 20 or more = score 3)
- Necrosis (absent = score 0, less than 50% of the tumour = score 1, more than 50% of the tumour = score 2)
- Grade **1** = scores 2–3, grade **2** = scores 4–5, grade **3** = scores 6–7

Lipomatous tumours form a significant bulk of the benign and malignant tumours assessed.

The commonest benign tumours are:
- Lipoma
- Spindle cell lipoma
- Angiolipoma
- Giant cell tumour of the tendon sheath
- Haemangioma
- Vascular leiomyoma
- Neurofibroma
- Schwannoma

The commonest malignant tumours encountered are:
- Liposarcoma
- Leiomyosarcoma
- Myxoid liposarcoma
- Synovial sarcoma
- Ewing's sarcoma
- Pleomorphic sarcoma NOS

Fluorescence in-situ hybridisation (FISH) plays a crucial role in evaluating adipocytic tumours. The presence of **MDM2 amplification** confirms the diagnosis of liposarcoma (Figure 13.1).

FISH studies are also commonly carried out to confirm:
- Myxoid liposarcoma: **DDIT3**
- Synovial sarcoma: **SS18**
- Spindle cell lipoma: **RB1**
- Ewing's sarcoma: **EWSR-1-FLI-1**

There are numerous other FISH probes which can be used depending on the clinical, morphological and immunohistochemical characteristics.

Mutational analysis and RNA fusion panel studies are other methods of molecular analysis of soft tissue tumours.

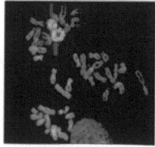

Ring (12)

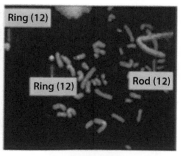

Rods and rings

Figure 13.1: MDM2 amplification in well-differentiated liposarcoma – home grown RD11-450G15 clone.

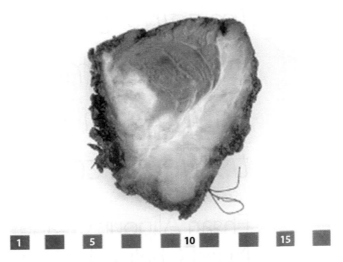

Figure 13.2: Resection of ill-defined tumour present at margins.

RESECTION OF SOFT TISSUE TUMOURS

Following image-guided biopsies, resections are carried out depending on the histopathological diagnosis and the anatomical location of the tumour. The tumour can reach the resection margins, as seen in Figure 13.2.

The margins of clearance are measured in millimetres. Complete excision of malignant tumours is anticipated as far as possible, depending on the plane of sections.

Take-home points

- It is essential to provide detailed clinical history and key imaging findings in pathology requests.
- MDTM discussion is recommended and can be particularly helpful in cases where there may be discrepancies between pathology and radiology.
- Cytogenetics (FISH) plays a vital role in the evaluation of several soft tissue lesions.

SUGGESTED READING

- Goldblum JR, Weiss SW, Folpe AL. Enzinger and Weiss's soft tissue tumors E-book. Elsevier Health Sciences; 2013 Oct 11.

14 Imaging of post-treatment changes in soft tissue sarcomas

Ehsan Alipour, Oganes Ashikyan,
Majid Chalian, Parham Pezeshk

INTRODUCTION

Soft tissue sarcomas (STS) are a diverse group of malignancies originating from mesenchymal tissues. The incidence of STS is estimated to be about 6 in 100,000 or about 1% of all cancers. It is important to note that out of all tumours originating in connective tissues, only about 10% are malignant.

Recent advances in diagnostic and therapeutic methods have made timely diagnosis and treatment possible for many sarcomas. In fact, the 5-year survival rate of STS has reached about 60%. The mainstay of STS treatment is surgical excision. Sometimes reconstructive surgeries are required to fill in the large defects remaining after resection. It is important to achieve clear margins on initial excision as it is an important predictor of remission. Studies have shown that positive microscopic margins after surgery highly correlate with local recurrence. Radiotherapy is also commonly used as both neo-adjuvant and adjuvant therapy for STS. Neo-adjuvant therapy facilitates surgical excision and increases the chance of clear margins. However, post-surgical complications are more common when radiotherapy is used. The role of chemotherapy as neo-adjuvant or adjuvant therapy is controversial, and it is only used in some high-risk patients. However, in metastatic disease, palliative chemotherapy is considered as the main treatment.

Imaging is the initial modality of choice to evaluate soft tissue lesions and is followed by tissue sampling in indeterminate or malignant cases. Magnetic resonance imaging (MRI) provides the best diagnostic information when it comes to sarcomas in extremities, trunk and pelvis (Figure 14.1). Computed tomography (CT) can help when there is contraindication for MRI or when the lesion is retroperitoneal. Radiography has limited diagnostic yield in the evaluation of STS; however, it could be helpful to assess the calcifications within the lesion which narrows the differential diagnosis. Meanwhile, it could be used to search for bone lesions. Ultrasonography (US) has value in triaging superficial palpable lesions but proven STS mostly need MRI to further characterise the lesion and the extent of subjacent tissue involvement.

DOI: 10.1201/9781003218722-14

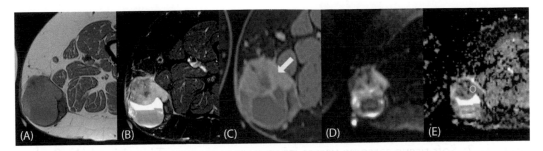

Figure 14.1: Use of advance MRI in the suspected sarcoma. Lobulated and heterogeneous soft tissue mass in the posteromedial aspect of the left thigh on T1-weighted (A), T2-weighted fat-suppressed (B), post-contrast subtraction (C), and diffusion-weighted images including B400 (D) and ADC map (E). Images demonstrate a heterogeneous mass with enhancing solid component (yellow arrow in E) and ADC value of 7.6 Å~10^{-3} mm²/s (yellow circle in E). Histologically proven pleomorphic sarcoma.

THE RADIOLOGICAL CHALLENGE

Local recurrence (LR) is an issue that complicates the treatment of STS. It is estimated that between 17 and 26% of these cancers recur 5 years after curative treatment and this number climbs up to as high as 32% in 10 years. Among STS, those that are truncal and in deep retroperitoneum (please refer to Figure 3.8 in Chapter 3), neck or head regions are more prone to local recurrence. Timely diagnosis of local recurrence can result in better outcomes for the patient. Routine periodic clinical and imaging evaluation help early detection of local recurrence. However, given that most patients undergo surgery and radiotherapy, normal anatomy is distorted and post-surgical changes and complications like scar tissue formation, hematomas and seromas can all complicate diagnosis of recurrence versus expected post-surgical changes or non-malignant complications. In this chapter, we will discuss the best practices in radiologic follow up of STS patients for timely and accurate LR detection.

IMAGING MODALITIES USED IN FOLLOW UP OF PATIENTS WITH STS

● *Ultrasound*

Ultrasound is used by some professionals along with physical examination as it is affordable and accessible. It serves as a useful screening modality differentiating post-operative seroma, haematoma or infection from LR. However, the US is operator dependent and its non-specific findings may require further characterisation by MRI.

● *Magnetic resonance imaging*

MRI is the preferred modality of choice for post-surgical follow up.

Studies show that using advanced MRI sequences such as diffusion-weighted imaging (DWI) (Figure 14.2) and dynamic contrast enhancement (DCE) techniques (Figure 14.3) in addition to conventional MRI can improve the diagnostic accuracy for post-treatment assessment of STS and aid differentiation between expected post-surgery imaging appearances and

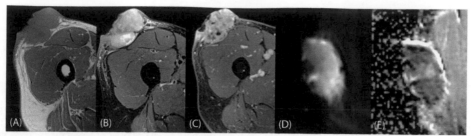

Figure 14.2: Soft tissue sarcoma verses inflammatory changes. T1-weighted (A), fluid-sensitive (B), post-contrast (C) and diffusion-weighted sequences (D and E) demonstrate a lobulated and heterogeneously enhancing soft tissue mass centred at subcutaneous fat of the anterior thigh with overlying ulceration. Heterogenous tumour enhancement clinches the diagnosis as abscesses usually show peripheral rim enhancement. Restricted diffusion would be equivocal in differentiating the abscess from ulcerated sarcoma with surrounding inflammatory changes.

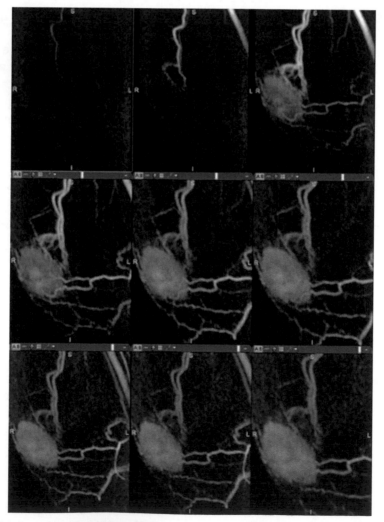

Figure 14.3: Utility of DCE-MRI in recurrent sarcoma. Dynamic contrast-enhanced (DCE) MRI with sequential images acquired every 5 seconds demonstrates enhancement of the mass from early arterial phase of contrast injection. Rapid arterial enhancement is a sign of high vascularity and could be a concerning finding in soft tissue masses.

recurrence. MRI has a sensitivity of 98% and specificity of 90% for LR and advantages of high-contrast resolution and multiplanar capability.

Limitations of MRI include field distortion artefacts at the region of concern if metal prostheses have been used and standard MRI contraindications such as pacemakers and cochlear implants.

● *Nuclear imaging*

Positron emission tomography-computed tomography (PET-CT) is also used for detection of LR and is recommended as a complementary method when MRI alone is hard to interpret (please refer to Figure 8.9 in Chapter 8).

PET-CT has the advantage of imaging the whole body and searching for distant metastasis.

In addition, factors like infectious disease or use of granulocyte colony-stimulating factor (G-CSF) can cause false positives in PET-CT and this imaging modality exposes patients to ionizing radiation.

If the primary tumour shows uptake on PET, PET-CT can be used to help with diagnoses of LR and distant metastasis in STS.

● *Chest radiographs and CT scan*

Chest radiograph or chest CT is used in follow up of patients with STS to rule out lung involvement (Figure 14.4). Radiographs have poor soft tissue visualisation and are not recommended as a screening imaging for LR in STS patients apart from lung metastases screening.

EXPECTED POST-TREATMENT CHANGES IN STS

Non-malignant post-treatment changes can be categorised into two groups: normal physiologic changes (e.g. oedema, granulation tissues and fibrosis) and complications (such as hematoma and post-operative seroma; Chart 14.1). In the following section, we will discuss the imaging findings of these changes. It should also be noted that if the patient undergoes radiotherapy, these changes may be more conspicuous and persistent. It is crucial to review the pre-treatment MRI of the STS to gather information regarding the signal characteristics, location, enhancement pattern and involvement of the subjacent structures.

● *Post-treatment changes*

Post-radiation oedema: Depending on the type of radiation, oedema-like signal, which is hyperintense on fluid-sensitive sequences such as T2-weighted, STIR (short-tau inversion recovery), or proton density fat-saturation (PDFS) sequences can persist for 6–18 months and in some cases may never completely resolve (Figures 14.8F–H).

Post-treatment tissue changes, scarring and hypertrophy: Collagenous septations can form in the subcutaneous tissue demonstrating alternating soft tissue and fluid-like signals. Signal characteristics following the fluid are more diffuse in the muscle. Histologically, the tissue structure is intact creating a feather-like appearance. The key feature differentiating the

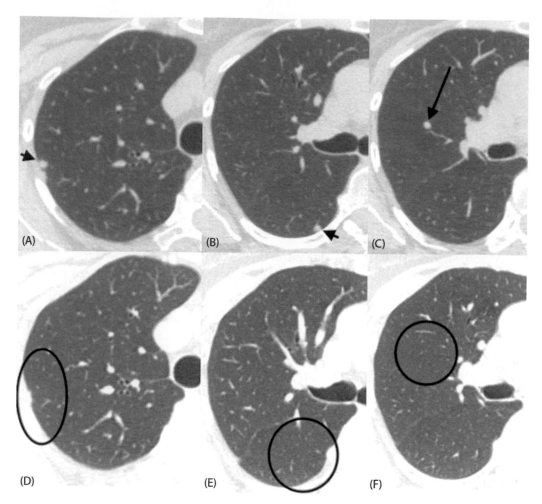

Figure 14.4: Use of the high-resolution CT (HRCT) in detecting lung metastases. Axial HRCT images (A–C) demonstrate newly developed subpleural and parenchymal nodules (black arrows) four months after the initial scan (D–F) performed as a part of staging CT in a patient with synovial sarcoma undergoing neo-adjuvant radiotherapy. The patient showed progression of the disease despite the therapy cycles due to interval development of distant metastatic disease and progressive local disease superimposed on post-radiotherapy changes. (Image Courtesy of Dr Siddharth Thaker.)

post-treatment changes from progressive disease is absent/minimal contrast enhancement (Figure 14.5). Intermuscular septa and adipose tissue may show hypertrophy eventually but increased contrast uptake should not be seen.

Post-surgical scar: A hypointense fibrose tissue could form at the surgical bed (Figure 14.5). The fibrotic tissue formed after surgery might be large (hypertrophied scar) and might even show nodular enhancement. The scar size is often proportional to the size of the tissue removed during the surgery and scar tissue usually does not show significant extension beyond margins. The diagnosis of recurrence in the setting of fibrosis and granulation tissues can be very challenging. Early arterial enhancement on the DCE sequence, which was found to be 100% sensitive

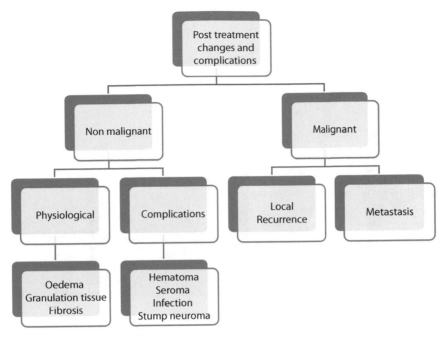

Chart 14.1: Post-treatment changes and complications seen in soft tissue sarcoma treatment. (Chart contributed by Dr Harun Gupta, Consultant Musculoskeletal Radiologist, Leeds Teaching Hospitals, Leeds, UK.)

and 97% specific in one study, when used with surrogate changes such as fatty marrow conversion in the irradiated bone. Imaging-guided biopsy and histological evaluation is recommended if the clinical dilemma persists.

● *Post-treatment complications*

Post-treatment complications that could be diagnosed with imaging include infection, seroma, hematoma, flap failure and necrosis (please refer to Figure 8.9 in Chapter 8). Radiation

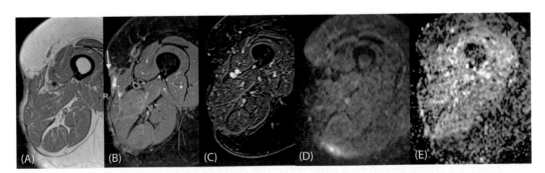

Figure 14.5: Expected post-surgical changes (scarring). Soft tissue defect in the medial aspect of the left thigh with scarring and no mass in T1-weighed (A) and fluid-sensitive (B) sequences. No nodular enhancement in subtraction post-contrast image (C) to suggest tumour recurrence. Diffusion-weighted images including B400 (D) and ADC map (E) show no focus of restriction.

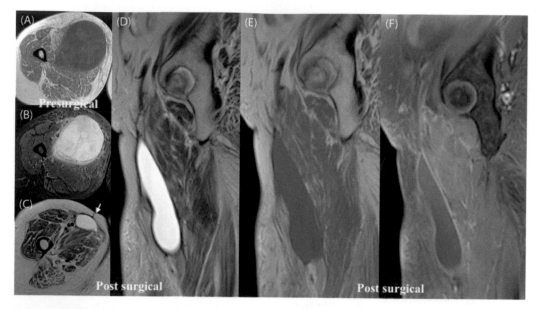

Figure 14.6: Post-operative seroma: The patient has had surgical excision for myxoid liposarcoma (A and B) in the medial compartment of the right thigh presented with a new fluctuant swelling under the excision scar (white arrow) which showed a wall-off collection following fluid intensity on T2-weight axial (C) and sagittal (D) and T1-weighted sagittal (E) images. It demonstrated thin enhancing pseudo-wall (F) following gadolinium administration consistent with seroma. No enhancing soft tissue component was seen within the lesion. (Image Courtesy of Dr Siddharth Thaker.)

therapy, especially neo-adjuvant radiation therapy, can increase the chances of these complications as well.

Post-operative seromas: They are well-marginated fluid collections that demonstrate simple homogenous non-enhancing hyperintense T2 signal. Their thin pseudo-capsule usually demonstrates thin peripheral enhancement (Figure 14.6). Depending on their protein and hemosiderin content, they might have variable signal intensity on T1-weighted sequences. Seromas may contain debris and usually regress within 3 to 18 months.

Post-operative haematomas: They appear as heterogenous cystic areas at the resection sites. Due to their hemosiderin content, they can show blooming artefact on gradient-echo (GRE) sequences. They might show minimal contrast uptake especially if they are chronic in nature. Hematomas change in shape and size as time passes by. Chronic expanding hematoma, a rarer entity, may be confused with LR. Sometimes a biopsy is necessary to differentiate between the two conditions.

Infections and abscesses: They are occasional after surgical resection of the tumours. Abscesses are characterised by a cystic structure demonstrating hyperintensity on STIR and other fluid-sensitive sequences and hypo- to isointense signal on T1-weighted sequence depending upon its contents. They may show peripheral rim enhancement if the gadolinium is used. The imaging interpretation is generally aided by a clinical picture of the sepsis. Imaging findings of abscesses, hematomas and recurrent necrotic neoplasms may overlap and further sampling may be needed to differentiate them.

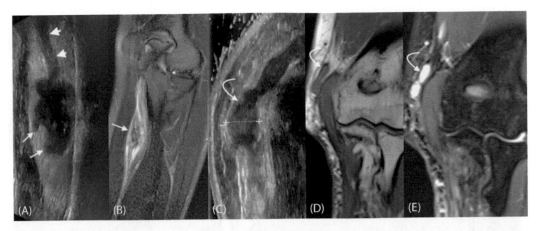

Figure 14.7: Stump neuroma: Greyscale ultrasound (A) and T2-weighted fat-suppressed coronal MRI (B) images showed irregular solid aggressive mass lesion (white arrows) within the flexor muscle compartment at the proximal forearm level. On ultrasound, the ulnar nerve (white arrowheads) can be seen entering into the lesion. The lesion proved to be an epitheliod sarcoma with neural involvement. Please appreciate neurogenic fatty and oedematous changes within the ulnar head of the flexor carpi ulnaris muscle. The lesion was excised with wide margins and ulnar nerve was sacrificed till elbow with clear nerve margins on histology. The patient represented with a posteromedial elbow swelling and neural pain. Greyscale ultrasound image (C) showed smooth bulbous enlargement of the ulnar nerve stump (compare ultrasound appearance of original tumour and stump neuroma) which did not show any aggressive features on T1-weighted (D) and STIR (E) MRI images. (Image Courtesy of Dr. Harun Gupta.)

Inflammatory pseudotumours: They are uncommon and occur following radiotherapy in 5 to 12.5% of cases with a substantial time lag (median time is around five years). These lesions are generally small, oval-shaped and heterogeneous. To distinguish them from LR, DCE imaging could be performed and time to contrast uptake should be reviewed. While in recurrences uptake is usually rapid and within 1 to 2 minutes of the administration of contrast, pseudotumour uptake is delayed and can happen 3 to 9 minutes later.

Stump neuromas: Nerves can undergo changes due to either recurrence or fibrosis. These changes are usually manifested as innervation oedema. In addition, neuromas might form at the size of resection (Figure 14.7).

TUMOR RESPONSE TO THERAPY

Sarcoma team and radiologists rely upon imaging to assess tumour response and progression when neo-adjuvant therapy is performed or when total resection is not technically possible. Factors like tumour size, necrosis and perfusion can determine the response of tumour to the therapy. To determine necrosis, reduced enhancement and perfusion are taken into account. Some studies show that to be considered successful, at least 90% of necrosis needs to be seen after neo-adjuvant therapy. It is also expected that the tumour shrinks in size following radiotherapy or chemotherapy. However, size criteria are ambiguous and could be misleading when assessing treatment response. Histopathological changes such as inflammation, necrosis, cystic change, haemorrhage, hyalinisation and fibrosis, which occur following neo-adjuvant therapy may influence size-based response assessment significantly (Figure 14.8).

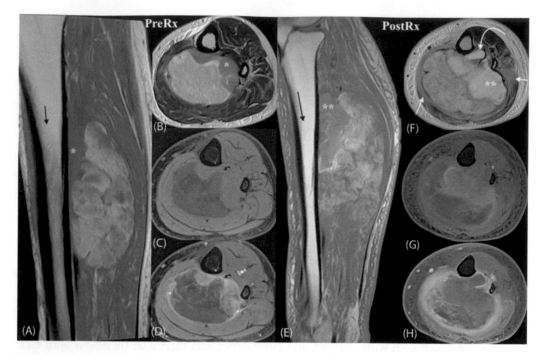

Figure 14.8: Local progression of the synovial sarcoma intermixed with post-radiotherapy changes: Pre-radiotherapy images – (A) T1-weighted sagittal and (B) T2-weighted axial MRI images showed a large soft tissue mass lesion involving the deep posterior muscle compartment of the left leg. There is preservation of the patchy red marrow in the tibial shaft (black arrow). The lesion showed aggressive appearances with mixed fatty and soft tissue component (asterisk) which demonstrated intense enhancement following gadolinium administration (C and D). Post-radiotherapy images – (E) T1-weighted sagittal and (F) T2-weighted axial MRI images showing fatty marrow replacement (black arrow), increased mass dimensions and effect, increased T1-weighted and T2-weighted signal in deep soft tissue component (double asterisk) which did not enhance post-contrast images (G and H) consistent with haemorrhagic transformation following radiotherapy, fatty component is also enlarged in the interim showing patchy contrast enhancement. Newly developed cystic component depicted fluid-haemorrhage level (curved arrow) with fluid leakage through interosseous septum into the anterior compartment. Extensive subcutaneous fat and muscle (straight arrows) oedema with contrast enhancement consistent with radiotherapy-related changes. (Image Courtesy of Dr Siddharth Thaker.)

● *Signs of progressive disease and local recurrence*

LR are mostly similar to the original tumour in terms of signal intensity and pattern of enhancement. Therefore, to detect LR, the radiologist should review the initial pre-treatment and prior post-treatment imagings. LRs are usually hyperintense on fluid-sensitive sequences and are mass like with nodular enhancement. So, any new growth at the site of resection or in adjacent tissues along the margins of surgical site should prompt further investigation (Figure 14.9).

New growth should be followed and assessed with contrast imaging. LR tend to have early uptake of contrast. It is important to note that early on, the granulation tissue can also have

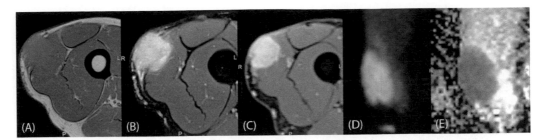

Figure 14.9: 58-year-old patient with local recurrence of soft tissue sarcoma. T1-weighted (A), fluid-sensitive (B), post-contrast (C) and DWI sequences show a heterogeneously enhancing mass with fascia and muscle invasion and restricted diffusion (D and E).

a high early uptake of contrast material. But this high uptake subsides after up to six months. Another sign specific to LR is detection of arterial flooding on the DCE sequence. In addition, diffusion restriction on DWI sequence with low apparent diffusion co-efficient (ADC) can be a sign of LR. Low ADC is correlated with high cellularity and is more often seen in LR than fibrosis or granulation tissue. Inflammatory pseudotumours also can have low ADC values but are rare. Nevertheless, low ADC is considered to be a specific sign for recurrence.

● *Therapy-related changes unique to myxoid liposarcoma*

Some tumours might not behave as expected in the post-treatment imaging. For example, myxoid liposarcoma does not always have contrast uptake on gadolinium-enhanced MRI and usually not avid on the PET/CT. They may show reduction in the myxoid component, seen as reduction in the hyperintensity on STIR images and increase in the fat signal on T1-weighted images, if neo-adjuvant radiotherapy is used (Figure 14.10). Such examples highlight the importance of knowledge about the primary tumour before attempting to rule out local recurrence.

Radiation-induced sarcoma: They can occur in both bone and soft tissue following at least 50 Gy of radiation after usually an extended period of time. These tumours are usually high-grade, and the most common subtype is malignant fibrous histiocytoma. Post-radiation sarcoma should be treated as new tumours and their prognosis depends on their size and grading.

Take-home points:

- Post-treatment baseline and follow-up imaging is required to assess recurrence. MRI offers the highest sensitivity and specify for this purpose. Other imaging modalities such as CT scan or PET/CT can be used to assess metastasis.
- It is crucial to review the treatment history as well as initial and prior imaging. Most of the time, a recurrence will resemble the original tumour so familiarity with the initial imagining findings of the tumour is of paramount importance. Non-malignant findings include oedema, collagenous septations, seroma, hematoma, pseudotumours, infections and hypertrophic scars. With respect to hematoma, sometimes it is hard to distinguish from LR as it can take up contrast and grow over time. In addition, pseudotumours can pose a challenge as they have low ADC values and could appear later on follow up.

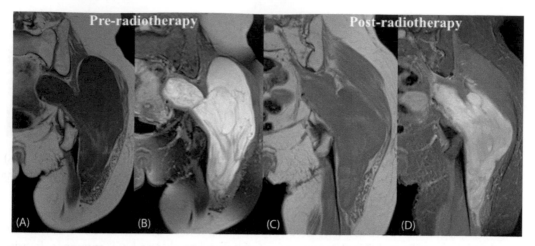

Figure 14.10: Post-radiotherapy changes in the myxoid liposarcoma (treatment response): T1-weighted (A) and STIR (B) images demonstrated a large soft tissue mass involving the left gluteal muscle compartment extending into the left hemipelvis through the obturator foramen. The lesion was diagnosed as myxoid liposarcoma on histology. Comparable post-radiotherapy (C) T1-weighted and STIR (D) images showed marked tumour shrinkage especially the hemipelvis and superior gluteal component. The myxoid component has also decreased with fatty areas becoming more conspicuous on T1-weighted image (C). (Image Courtesy of Dr Siddharth Thaker.)

- When a tumour responds to therapy, we expect this response to be in the form of necrosis and shrinkage in size. There are exceptions to this rule as discussed above. Necrosis can be manifested by reduction in contrast intake and perfusion.
- Local recurrence is usually in the form of nodular enhancement which usually follows the pattern of the original tumour.
- A small percentage of recurrences are tumours that occur due to radiotherapy. These can happen in bone and soft tissue at later stages on follow up.

SUGGESTED READING

- Bloem, JL, Vriens, D, Krol, ADG, Özdemir, M, Sande, MAJ van de, Gelderblom, H, et al. Therapy-related imaging findings in patients with sarcoma. Semin Musculoskelet Radiol. 2020 Dec;24(06):676–691.
- England, P, Hong, Z, Rhea, L, Hirbe, A, McDonald, D, Cipriano, C. Does advanced imaging have a role in detecting local recurrence of soft-tissue sarcoma? Clin Orthop Relat Res. 2020 Dec;478(12):2812–2820.
- Ezuddin, NS, Pretell-Mazzini, J, Yechieli, RL, Kerr, DA, Wilky, BA, Subhawong, TK. Local recurrence of soft-tissue sarcoma: Issues in imaging surveillance strategy. Skelet Radiol. 2018 Dec;47(12):1595–1606.
- Garner, HW, Kransdorf, MJ, Bancroft, LW, Peterson, JJ, Berquist, TH, Murphey, MD. Benign and malignant soft-tissue tumors: Posttreatment MR imaging. Radiographics. 2009 Jan;29(1):119–134.
- Gennaro, N, Reijers, S, Bruining, A, Messiou, C, Haas, R, Colombo, P, et al. Imaging response evaluation after neoadjuvant treatment in soft tissue sarcomas: Where do we stand? Crit Rev Oncol/Hematol. 2021 Apr;160:103309.
- Noebauer-Huhmann, I-M, Chaudhary, SR, Papakonstantinou, O, Panotopoulos, J, Weber, M-A, Lalam, RK, et al. Soft tissue sarcoma follow-up imaging: Strategies to distinguish post-treatment changes from recurrence. Semin Musculoskelet Radiol. 2020 Dec;24(06):627–644.
- Park, JW, Yoo, HJ, Kim, H-S, Choi, J-Y, Cho, HS, Hong, SH, et al. MRI surveillance for local recurrence in extremity soft tissue sarcoma. Eur J Surg Oncol. 2019 Feb;45(2):268–274.
- Soldatos, T, Ahlawat, S, Montgomery, E, Chalian, M, Jacobs, MA, Fayad, LM. Multiparametric assessment of treatment response in high-grade soft-tissue sarcomas with anatomic and functional MR imaging sequences. Radiology. 2016 Mar;278(3):831–840.

Index

Note: Locators in *italics* represent figures and **bold** indicate tables in the text.